USER'S GUIDE FOR THE

SCID-5-CV

STRUCTURED CLINICAL INTERVIEW

FOR DSM-5® DISORDERS

CLINICIAN VERSION

USER'S GUIDE FOR THE

SCID-5-CV

STRUCTURED CLINICAL INTERVIEW
FOR DSM-5® DISORDERS

CLINICIAN VERSION

Michael B. First, M.D.
Professor of Clinical Psychiatry, Columbia University, and Research Psychiatrist,
Division of Clinical Phenomenology, New York State Psychiatric Institute,
New York, New York

Janet B.W. Williams, Ph.D.
Professor Emerita of Clinical Psychiatric Social Work (in Psychiatry and in
Neurology), Columbia University, and Research Scientist and Deputy Chief,
Biometrics Research Department (Retired), New York State Psychiatric Institute,
New York, New York; and Senior Vice President of Global Science,
MedAvante, Inc., Hamilton, New Jersey

Rhonda S. Karg, Ph.D.
Research Psychologist, Division of Behavioral Health and
Criminal Justice Research, RTI International, Durham, North Carolina

Robert L. Spitzer, M.D.
Professor Emeritus of Psychiatry, Columbia University, and
Research Scientist and Chief, Biometrics Research Department (Retired),
New York State Psychiatric Institute, New York, New York

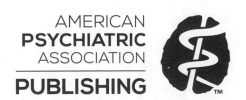

AMERICAN
PSYCHIATRIC
ASSOCIATION
PUBLISHING

Manufactured in the United States of America on acid-free paper
23   22   21   7   6

Typeset in Palatino and Futura.

American Psychiatric Association Publishing
800 Maine Ave. SW
Suite 900
Washington, DC 20024-2812
www.appi.org

Contents

Acknowledgments

We thank Desiree Caban, our research assistant and all-round jack-of-all-trades at Biometrics Research at Columbia University, for all of her invaluable assistance in helping to manage this project.

Drafts of the SCID-5 were made available to experienced SCID users, who reviewed these drafts and provided extremely helpful suggestions. We also sought consultation with a number of DSM-5 Work Group members. We gratefully acknowledge the following contributors for their invaluable assistance in developing the SCID-5:

John J.B. Allen	University of Arizona
Emily Ansell	Yale University School of Medicine
Martin M. Antony	Ryerson University
Cathie Atkinson	Institute of Behavioral Medicine Research, Ohio State University
Evelyn Attia	Columbia University
Deanna Barch	Washington University, St. Louis
Arthur Barsky	Harvard University
Stephen Benning	University of Nevada, Las Vegas
Melanie Biggs	VA North Texas Health Care System, Dallas VA Medical Center, and University of Texas, Southwestern Medical Center at Dallas
Cheryl Birch	Jett Psychological Services
Ryan Blazei	RTI International
J. Alexander Bodkin	Harvard University, McLean Hospital
Juan Manuel Bravo Sierra	CETTAD, Mexico City
Benjamin B. Brody	TeleSage Health Outcomes, Inc.
Rachel Bryant-Waugh	Great Ormond Street Hospital NHS Foundation Trust
Juan Bustillo	University of New Mexico
Amanda Calkins	Massachusetts General Hospital
William Carpenter	University of Maryland
Kathleen M. Chard	Cincinnati Veterans Administration Medical Center
Seema Clifasefi	University of Washington, Harborview Medical Center
Emil F. Coccaro	University of Chicago
Susan E. Collins	University of Washington, Harborview Medical Center
Michelle Craske	University of California, Los Angeles
Daniel David	Babeş-Bolyai University
Joanne Davis	University of Tulsa
Joel Dimsdale	University of California, San Diego
Aubrey Enloe	MedAvante, Inc.
Beth Epstein	Rutgers University
Sophia Frangou	Icahn School of Medicine at Mount Sinai

Ellen Frank	University of Pittsburgh
Stephenie Frank	University of Oregon
Matthew J. Friedman	National Center for PTSD, U.S. Department of Veterans Affairs, Geisel School of Medicine at Dartmouth
Wolfgang Gaebel	University of Dusseldorf
Jon Grant	University of Chicago
Raquel Gur	University of Pennsylvania Medical Center
Gretchen L. Haas	University of Pittsburgh
Glenn Haley	Timber Creek Tertiary Mental Health Program
Stephan Heckers	Vanderbilt University School of Medicine
David Hellerstein	Columbia University Medical Center
Jörgen Herlofson	Pilgrim Press
Peter J. Kelly	University of Wollongong
Ronald C. Kessler	Harvard Medical School
Daniel Klein	Stony Brook University
Rachel Klein	New York University Langone Medical Center
Anna Kokkevi	Athens University Medical School, University Mental Health Research Institute
Frances Levin	Columbia University
Dolores Malaspina	New York University Langone Medical Center
David Mataix-Cols	Karolinska Institutet, Stockholm, Sweden
Michael McCloskey	Temple University
Giovani Missio	Vitzlmente Institute
Parvaneh Mohammadkhani	University of Social Welfare and Rehabilitation Sciences, Iran
Debra M. Montrose	Western Psychiatric Institute and Clinic
Antonia S. New	Mount Sinai Hospital
Karen Nolan	Nathan S. Kline Institute for Psychiatric Research and New York University Lagone Medical Center
Mary O'Brien	Yale University
Felice Ockun	MedAvante, Inc.
Michael J. Owen	Cardiff University School of Medicine
Kate Panzer	Kate Panzer Consulting
Rosanna Perone	Associazione Italiana per la cura delle Dipendenze Patologiche Azienda USL 10, Firenze, Italy
Kate Peruzzini	Harvard University
Katharine Phillips	Brown University
Michael R. Phillips	Shanghai Mental Health Center and Emory University
Agnieszka Popiel	University of Social Sciences and Humanities, Warsaw, Poland
Charles F. Reynolds, III	University of Pittsburgh
Jane Roberts	University of South Carolina
Ruth Rozensztejn	OSDE Argentina

Lesia Ruglass	The City College of New York
Sanjaya Saxena	University of California, San Diego
Brad Schmidt	Florida State University
Nina Schooler	State University of New York Downstate Medical Center
Susan K. Schulz	University of Iowa
Robert Schütze	School of Psychology and Speech Pathology, Curtin University
Daniel L. Segal	University of Colorado, Colorado Springs
Stewart Shankman	University of Illinois at Chicago
Katherine Sharkey	Brown University, Alpert Medical School
Brian A. Sharpless	Washington State University
H. Blair Simpson	Columbia University Medical Center
Roxanna Snaauw	RTI International
Murray Stein	University of California, San Diego
Trisha Suppes	Stanford University School of Medicine
Julianna Switaj	Norfolk Psychological Services, College of Psychologists at Ontario
Sumner Jay Sydeman	Northern Arizona University
Rajiv Tandon	University of Florida
Charles Tapp	Raphah Counselling
Kathleen Torsney	William Paterson University
Timothy Trull	University of Missouri at Columbia
Jim Van Os	Maastricht University
Vytas Velyvis	CBT Associates of Toronto, Adler Institute, University Health Network
Elaine Veracruz	Harvard University
B. Timothy Walsh	Columbia University Medical School
Joris Wiggers	Vancouver Island Health Authority
Hans-Ulrich Wittchen	Dresden University
Justyna Zapolska	The City University of New York, John Jay College of Criminal Justice
Mark Zimmerman	Brown University, Alpert Medical School

We would like to give special thanks to the following colleagues for their especially extensive input: Dusty Hackler (Teachers College, Columbia University, New York State Psychiatric Institute); Jenny Jordon (University of Otago, Christchurch, New Zealand); Rudolf Uher (Dalhousie University); Catherine Dempsey (Uniformed Services University of the Health Sciences); and the SCID interviewers at the Henry Jackson Foundation (Mary Schumann, George Mason University; Shayne Power, Uniformed Services University of the Health Sciences; and Patricia Spangler, Uniformed Services University of the Health Sciences) for their help in trying out drafts of the SCID-5 over the past 2 years.

Finally, we would like to thank those at American Psychiatric Association Publishing who assisted in the production of the SCID-5-CV: Robert E. Hales, M.D., Editor-in-Chief; Rebecca Rinehart, Publisher; John McDuffie, Associate Publisher; Susan Westrate, Production Manager, for the careful typesetting of all elements and the cover and book design; Patricia Freedman, for her careful proofreading; and especially Ann M. Eng, Senior Developmental Editor, whose meticulous and thoughtful editing helped ensure that the various details of this complex instrument fit together seamlessly.

Citation and Additional Copyright Notices

For citation: First MB, Williams JBW, Karg RS, Spitzer RL: *User's Guide for the Structured Clinical Interview for DSM-5 Disorders—Clinician Version (SCID-5-CV).* Arlington, VA, American Psychiatric Association, 2016

The Structured Clinical Interview for DSM-5® Disorders—Clinician Version (SCID-5-CV) comprises this User's Guide and the SCID-5-CV interview booklet (each sold separately). No part of these publications may be photocopied, reproduced, stored in a retrieval system, or transmitted, in any form or by any means, without obtaining permission in writing from American Psychiatric Association Publishing, or as expressly permitted by law, by license, or by terms agreed with the appropriate reproduction rights organization. All such inquiries, including those concerning reproduction outside the scope of the above, should be sent to Rights Department, American Psychiatric Association Publishing, 1000 Wilson Blvd., Suite 1825, Arlington, VA 22209-3901 or via the online permissions form at: http://www.appi.org/permissions. For more information, please visit the SCID products page on www.appi.org.

DSM-5® diagnostic criteria are reprinted or adapted with permission from American Psychiatric Association: *Diagnostic and Statistical Manual of Mental Disorders,* Fifth Edition. Arlington VA, American Psychiatric Association, 2013. Copyright © 2013 American Psychiatric Association. Used with permission.

Unless authorized in writing by the American Psychiatric Association (APA), no part of the DSM-5® criteria may be reproduced or used in a manner inconsistent with the APA's copyright. This prohibition applies to unauthorized uses or reproductions in any form, including electronic applications. Correspondence regarding copyright permission for DSM-5 criteria should be directed to DSM Permissions, American Psychiatric Association Publishing, 1000 Wilson Boulevard, Suite 1825, Arlington, VA 22209-3901.

Homework cases in Appendix B, "Training," are adapted with permission from Spitzer RL, Gibbon M, Skodol AE, Williams JBW, First MB: *DSM-IV-TR Casebook: A Learning Companion to the Diagnostic and Statistical Manual of Mental Disorders,* Fourth Edition, Text Revision. Arlington, VA, American Psychiatric Publishing, 2002. Copyright © 2002. Used with permission.

Disclosures

The following author has declared all forms of support received within the 12 months prior to manuscript submittal that may represent a competing interest in relation to her work published in this volume, as follows:

Janet B.W. Williams, Ph.D., works full-time as the Senior Vice President of Global Science, MedAvante, Inc., a pharmaceuticals services company.

The following authors of this work have no competing interests to report:

Michael B. First, M.D.; Rhonda S. Karg, Ph.D.; Robert L. Spitzer, M.D.

1. Introduction

The Structured Clinical Interview for DSM-5 (SCID-5) is a semistructured interview guide for making the major DSM-5 diagnoses (formerly diagnosed on Axis I). It is administered by a clinician or trained mental health professional who is familiar with the DSM-5 classification and diagnostic criteria (American Psychiatric Association 2013). The interview subjects may be either psychiatric or general medical patients—or individuals who do not identify themselves as patients, such as subjects in a community survey of mental illness or family members of psychiatric patients. The language and diagnostic coverage make the SCID-5 most appropriate for use with adults (age 18 and over); but with slight modification to the wording of the questions, it may be used with adolescents. The average person should be able to understand the language of the SCID-5. Some individuals with severe cognitive impairment, agitation, or severe psychotic symptoms cannot be interviewed using the SCID-5. This should be evident in the first 10 minutes of the Overview, and in such a case the SCID-5 may be used instead as a diagnostic checklist and decision tree, with diagnostic information obtained from other sources.

The SCID-5 can be used in a variety of ways:

- **To ensure that all of the major DSM-5 diagnoses are systematically evaluated.** For example, the SCID is often used as part of intake procedures in clinical settings and to help insure a comprehensive forensic diagnostic evaluation.
- **To select a study population.** For example, in a study of the effectiveness of a treatment for depression, the SCID-5 can be used to insure that all of the study subjects have symptoms that meet the DSM-5 criteria for Major Depressive Disorder and that all of the subjects with a history of any Substance Use Disorder in the past 12 months are excluded.
- **To characterize a study population in terms of current and past psychiatric diagnoses.** For example, diagnostic data that are obtained using the SCID-5 interview can be used by researchers, practitioners, policy makers, and the general public who are interested in prevalence and incidence estimates of psychiatric disorders among certain populations (e.g., adults in the United States).
- **To improve interviewing skills of students in the mental health professions,** including psychiatry, psychology, psychiatric social work, and psychiatric nursing. For example, the SCID-5 can provide trainees with a repertoire of useful questions to elicit information from a patient that will be the basis for making judgments about the diagnostic criteria. Through repeated administrations of the SCID-5, students become familiar with the DSM-5 criteria and at the same time incorporate useful questions into their interviewing repertoire.

For the latest information about the SCID-5, including available translations, computer-assisted versions, training materials including videos and SCID knowledge examinations, and error corrections/revisions, please visit the SCID Web site: www.scid5.org.

2.   History of the SCID

The publication of DSM-III in 1980 revolutionized psychiatry with its inclusion of specified diagnostic criteria for virtually all of the mental disorders (American Psychiatric Association 1980). Before 1980 there were several sets of diagnostic criteria, such as the Feighner Criteria (Feighner et al. 1972) and the Research Diagnostic Criteria (RDC; Spitzer et al. 1978), as well as structured interviews designed to make diagnoses according to these systems (Endicott and Spitzer 1978; Helzer et al. 1981). In 1983, work started on the SCID as an instrument for making DSM-III diagnoses in response to the widespread adoption of the DSM-III criteria as the standard language for describing research subjects. The SCID incorporated several features not present in previous instruments that would facilitate its use in psychiatric research, such as the inclusion of an Overview section that allows the patient to describe the development of the current episode of illness, and a modular design enabling researchers to eliminate consideration of major diagnostic classes that are irrelevant to their studies.

In 1983, the National Institute of Mental Health recognized the need for a clinical diagnostic assessment procedure for making DSM-III diagnoses and issued a Request for Proposal to develop such a procedure. Based on pilot work with the SCID, a contract was awarded to further develop the instrument. In April 1985, the Biometrics Research Department at New York State Psychiatric Institute received a 2-year grant to field-test the SCID and to determine its reliability in several different clinical and nonclinical subject groups (Spitzer et al. 1992; Williams et al. 1992). Following the publication of the revised DSM-III (DSM-III-R; American Psychiatric Association 1987), the SCID for DSM-III-R was published by American Psychiatric Press in May 1990 (Spitzer et al. 1990a, 1990b).

Work on the DSM-IV (American Psychiatric Association 1994) revision of the SCID began in fall 1993. Draft versions of the revision were field-tested by interested researchers during the second half of 1994. A final version of the SCID for DSM-IV was produced in February 1996. Several revisions of the SCID followed, the most extensive of which was made in February 2001 when the SCID was updated for the DSM-IV Text Revision (DSM-IV-TR; American Psychiatric Association 2000).

Work on revising the SCID for DSM-5 began in 2012. The multitude of changes in the DSM-5 criteria sets (American Psychiatric Association 2013) required the development of many new SCID questions, as well as adjustments to the SCID algorithm. The opportunity was also taken to revisit all of the questions and make modifications in the wording even for criterion items that had not changed in DSM-5. Draft revisions were reviewed by DSM-5 Work Group members and experienced SCID users during the first half of 2013, and field-testing of the SCID-5 began in late 2013. The final version of the SCID for DSM-5 was submitted to American Psychiatric Association Publishing for publication in August 2014.

3. Versions of the SCID

The SCID was originally designed to be a single document that could be used by both researchers and clinicians. This involved making the SCID detailed enough to meet the needs of the research community, but still user-friendly enough for use by clinicians to enhance the reliability and validity of their diagnostic assessments. This duality of purpose ultimately created problems for researchers because a lot of potentially useful diagnostic information was left out of the DSM-III-R version of the SCID in order to keep it from becoming too cumbersome (e.g., most of the subtypes). However, many clinicians felt that the amount of detail that was included in the SCID still rendered it too long and complex. Moreover, it also became clear that for clinical trials in which the SCID was used to determine whether potential subjects' conditions meet the diagnostic inclusion and exclusion criteria for particular protocols, the standard research version included a lot of extraneous information that was not needed for clinical trials. Thus, the need also arose for a version of the SCID that could be tailored specifically to the inclusion/exclusion criteria for clinical trials.

To meet these divergent needs, the SCID-5 has been split into three separate versions: the **Clinician Version** (SCID-5-CV), which has been streamlined for use in clinical settings; the **Research Version** (SCID-5-RV), which includes a number of features intended to facilitate its use in research studies; and the **Clinical Trials Version** (SCID-5-CT), which is available for customization to conform to the inclusion/exclusion criteria for a specific clinical trial. Details about the three versions are provided below.

3.1 Clinician Version of the SCID (SCID-5-CV)

This User's Guide pertains specifically to the Clinician Version of the SCID (SCID-5-CV). The SCID-5-CV is published as a bound booklet by American Psychiatric Association Publishing and is an abridged and reformatted version of the SCID-5-RV that covers those diagnoses most commonly seen in clinical settings. Despite the "clinician" designation, the SCID-5-CV can be used in research settings as long as the disorders of particular interest to the researcher are among those included in the SCID-5-CV.

The SCID-5-CV differs from the SCID-5-RV in several ways. First, the specifiers included in the SCID-5-CV are limited to those that have an impact on the diagnostic coding. Thus, only the severity, psychosis, and remission specifiers for Bipolar Disorder and Major Depressive Disorder are included in the SCID-5-CV because these affect the choice of diagnostic code. Similarly, the Attention-Deficit/Hyperactivity Disorder (ADHD) presentation types (i.e., predominantly inattentive, predominantly hyperactive/impulsive, and combined) are included because they are also required to determine the diagnostic code. Second, the criteria sets for a number of disorders (e.g., Anorexia Nervosa, Hoarding Disorder) included in the SCID-5-RV do not appear in the SCID-5-CV and instead are replaced with screening questions for those disorders in Module I ("Screening for Other Current Disorders"). If the patient answers one of these questions in the affirmative, the clinician needs to follow up with an unstructured clinical assessment of the diagnostic requirements for that disorder. (To facilitate this process, the SCID-5-CV User's Guide includes the DSM-5 criteria sets for these disorders in Appendix A, and the SCID-5-CV includes references to both the page numbers for the corresponding criteria sets in Appendix A as well as the page numbers in DSM-5.) Finally, although most of the disorders in the SCID-5-RV are assessed for both current and lifetime time frames, the SCID-5-CV focuses largely on whether criteria are currently met, because the current clinical status of a disorder is most relevant for treatment decisions. The only disorders in the SCID-5-CV that also include a lifetime assessment are Major Depressive Disorder, Bipolar I and II Disorders, Schizophrenia Spectrum and Other Psychotic Disorders, Panic Disorder, and Posttraumatic Stress Disorder (PTSD).

3.2   Research Version of the SCID (SCID-5-RV)

As the most comprehensive version of the SCID, the SCID-5-RV contains more disorders than the Clinician Version and includes all of the subtypes and severity and course specifiers in the DSM-5. Moreover, a particularly important feature of the SCID-5-RV is its customizability, allowing the instrument to be tailored to meet the requirements of a particular study.

The SCID-5-RV comes in a standard "core" configuration that includes those disorders most researchers are likely to want to assess routinely for most studies, as well as an "enhanced" configuration that also includes the assessment of a number of optional disorders. To facilitate customization, the SCID-5-RV is not published as a bound volume, but instead the diagnostic modules are only available electronically as either 18 PDF files (which can be printed out by the researcher and "bound" together for ease of use) or as 18 Microsoft (MS) Word documents that can be modified by the researcher in order to remove unneeded elements (e.g., certain specifiers), alter the flow through the interview, or add additional scales (e.g., severity rating scales) of the researcher's choosing.

3.3   Clinical Trials Version of the SCID (SCID-5-CT)

Originally developed in partnership with i3 Research, the SCID-5-CT is a modified version of the SCID-5-RV that has been reformatted, streamlined, and optimized for use in clinical trials that incorporate typical inclusion and exclusion criteria. SCID-CT templates have been developed for clinical trials for treatments of Major Depressive Disorder, Bipolar Disorder, Schizophrenia, Generalized Anxiety Disorder, PTSD, and ADHD. An additional "exclusionary" SCID-5-CT has also been developed for situations in which the SCID is used primarily to exclude individuals with disorders listed in the exclusion criteria for the study (e.g., for drug indications not included in the SCID, like Major Neurocognitive Disorder). In order to produce a protocol-specific SCID-CT, the appropriate template must be customized to conform to the particular inclusion/exclusion criteria for the protocol. Visit www.scid5.org for more information on obtaining a commercial license and to arrange for protocol-specific customization of the SCID-CT.

4. SCID-5-CV Diagnostic Coverage and Time Frame

The SCID-5-CV is divided into 10 relatively self-contained diagnostic modules. Table 4–1 indicates the symptoms, episodes, and disorders that are included in each of the modules. As noted in the right-hand column of the table, there are various time frames that apply to the assessment of the disorders in the SCID-5-CV. In order to simplify the SCID for clinical use, many disorders in the SCID-5-CV are assessed only for the current time period, because that time frame is likely to be most clinically relevant for the purposes of treatment selection and management. These "current only" disorders include Persistent Depressive Disorder, Substance Use Disorders, Agoraphobia, Social Anxiety Disorder, Generalized Anxiety Disorder, Obsessive-Compulsive Disorder (OCD), ADHD, and Adjustment Disorder. Other disorders are evaluated for their presence during the patient's lifetime, and are accompanied by additional questions to determine whether criteria have also been met during the current month. These include Bipolar I Disorder, Bipolar II Disorder, Other Specified/Unspecified Bipolar Disorder, Major Depressive Disorder, Other Specified/Unspecified Depressive Disorder, all of the Schizophrenia Spectrum and Other Psychotic Disorders, Panic Disorder, and PTSD. Most of these disorders are defined according to symptoms or events that have occurred during the individual's lifetime (e.g., exposure to traumatic event in PTSD, history of recurrent unexpected panic attacks in Panic Disorder).

In contrast to the disorders mentioned above, which involve the clinician providing a rating for each diagnostic criterion, Mental Disorders Due to Another Medical Condition (e.g., Bipolar Disorder Due to Another Medical Condition) and Substance/Medication-Induced Mental Disorders (e.g., Substance/Medication-Induced Anxiety Disorder) are diagnosed in the SCID-5-CV without assessing the diagnostic criteria for these disorders. Instead, the diagnoses of Mental Disorder Due to Another Medical Condition and Substance/Medication-Induced Mental Disorder are made in the course of evaluating the criteria in the primary disorders that rule out a general medical condition (GMC) or substance/medication etiology—e.g., "the disturbance is not attributable to the physiological effects of a substance (e.g., a drug of abuse, a medication) or another medical condition." In those cases when the clinician rules out a primary psychiatric diagnosis because of a GMC or substance/medication etiology, the clinician is instructed to diagnose the appropriate Mental Disorder Due to Another Medical Condition or Substance/Medication-Induced Mental Disorder and to record the diagnosis and its ICD-10-CM diagnostic code on the SCID-5-CV Diagnostic Summary Score Sheet. Moreover, interview questions corresponding to the individual diagnostic criteria are not provided for the disorders listed in Module I (most of which are evaluated in the "enhanced" version of the SCID-5-RV). Screening questions from the SCID-5-RV are provided instead and, if answered affirmatively by the patient, the clinician needs to evaluate their potential presence clinically, based on consulting the corresponding DSM-5 criteria sets.

TABLE 4–1.   **Diagnostic coverage of the SCID-5-CV (with applicable time periods)**

Module	Contents	Time Period
Module A **Mood Episodes and Persistent Depressive Disorder**	Major Depressive Episode	Current (past month) and past
	Manic Episode	Current (past month) and past
	Hypomanic Episode	Current (past month) and past
	Persistent Depressive Disorder (formerly Dysthymic Disorder)	Current (past 2 years)
Module B **Psychotic and Associated Symptoms**	Delusions	Lifetime
	Hallucinations	Lifetime
	Disorganized speech	Lifetime
	Disorganized behavior	Lifetime
	Catatonic behavior	Lifetime
	Negative symptoms	Lifetime
Module C **Differential Diagnosis of Psychotic Disorders**	Schizophrenia	Current (past month) and past
	Schizophreniform Disorder	Current (past month) and past
	Schizoaffective Disorder	Current (past month) and past
	Delusional Disorder	Current (past month) and past
	Brief Psychotic Disorder	Current (past month) and past
	Other Specified/Unspecified Psychotic Disorder	Current (past month) and past (remission)
	Psychotic Disorder Due to Another Medical Condition (AMC)	Lifetime
	Substance/Medication-Induced Psychotic Disorder	Lifetime
Module D **Differential Diagnosis of Mood Disorders**	Bipolar I Disorder	Current (past month) and past (remission)
	Bipolar II Disorder	Current (past month) and past (remission)
	Other Specified/Unspecified Bipolar Disorder	Current (past month) and past (remission)
	Bipolar Disorder Due to AMC	Lifetime
	Substance/Medication-Induced Bipolar Disorder	Lifetime
	Major Depressive Disorder	Current (past month) and past (remission)
	Other Specified/Unspecified Depressive Disorder	Current (past month) and past (remission)
	Depressive Disorder Due to AMC	Lifetime
	Substance/Medication-Induced Depressive Disorder	Lifetime
Module E **Substance Use Disorders**	Alcohol Use Disorder	Current (past 12 months)
	Sedative, Hypnotic, or Anxiolytic Use Disorder	Current (past 12 months)
	Cannabis Use Disorder	Current (past 12 months)
	Stimulant Use Disorder	Current (past 12 months)
	Opioid Use Disorder	Current (past 12 months)
	Phencyclidine and Related Substance Use Disorder	Current (past 12 months)

TABLE 4–1. **Diagnostic coverage of the SCID-5-CV (with applicable time periods)** *(continued)*

Module	Contents	Time Period
Module E Substance Use Disorders *(continued)*	Other Hallucinogen Use Disorder	Current (past 12 months)
	Inhalant Use Disorder	Current (past 12 months)
	Other (or Unknown) Substance Use Disorder	Current (past 12 months)
Module F Anxiety Disorders	Panic Disorder	Current (past month) and past
	Agoraphobia	Current (past 6 months)
	Social Anxiety Disorder	Current (past 6 months)
	Generalized Anxiety Disorder	Current (past 6 months)
	Anxiety Disorder Due to AMC	Lifetime
	Substance/Medication-Induced Anxiety Disorder	Lifetime
Module G Obsessive-Compulsive Disorder and Posttraumatic Stress Disorder	Obsessive-Compulsive Disorder	Current (past month)
	Obsessive-Compulsive and Related Disorder Due to AMC	Lifetime
	Substance/Medication-Induced Obsessive-Compulsive and Related Disorder	Lifetime
	Posttraumatic Stress Disorder	Current (past month) and past
Module H Adult Attention-Deficit/Hyperactivity Disorder	Attention-Deficit/Hyperactivity Disorder	Current (past 6 months)
Module I Screening for Other Current Disorders	Premenstrual Dysphoric Disorder Specific Phobia Separation Anxiety Disorder Hoarding Disorder Body Dysmorphic Disorder Trichotillomania (Hair Pulling Disorder) Excoriation (Skin-Picking) Disorder Insomnia Disorder Hypersomnolence Disorder Anorexia Nervosa Bulimia Nervosa Binge-Eating Disorder Avoidant/Restrictive Food Intake Disorder Somatic Symptom Disorder Illness Anxiety Disorder Intermittent Explosive Disorder Gambling Disorder	*Note:* Although screening is for current disorders, diagnostic criteria are not provided for these disorders in the SCID-5-CV.
Module J Adjustment Disorder	Adjustment Disorder	Current (past 6 months)

5.   Basic Features of the SCID-5-CV

5.1   Overview

The SCID begins with an open-ended Overview of the present illness and past episodes of psychopathology before leading the clinician to systematically inquire about the presence or absence of particular DSM-5 criterion items. This Overview provides opportunities to hear the patient describe any difficulties in his or her own words and to collect information that may not be covered in the course of assessing specific diagnostic criteria (e.g., treatment history, social and occupational functioning, context of developing symptoms). By the end of the Overview, the clinician should have gathered enough information to formulate a list of tentative diagnoses to be ruled out or substantiated by the diagnostic modules.

5.2   Diagnostic Flow

The sequence of questions in the SCID-5-CV is designed to approximate the differential diagnostic process of an experienced clinician. As the interview progresses and the DSM-5 diagnostic criteria embedded in the SCID are assessed, the clinician is, in effect, continually testing diagnostic hypotheses. Note that for some disorders, the diagnostic criteria are not listed in the same order as in DSM-5, but have been reordered to make the SCID interview more efficient or user-friendly. For example, Criterion D for Schizophrenia is listed right after Criterion A to allow the clinician to skip out of Schizophrenia immediately if the temporal relationship between psychotic and mood symptoms is not consistent with a diagnosis of Schizophrenia.

5.3   Ratings

Although specific structured questions are provided to help elicit diagnostic information, it is important to keep in mind the fact that the **ratings in the SCID-5-CV reflect the presence or absence of the DSM-5 diagnostic criteria and not necessarily the patient's answers to the SCID questions.** Ratings in the SCID-5-CV are as follows and are defined further in Section 7.4, "Ratings of Criterion Items" in this User's Guide:

—   = **Absent/subthreshold** (for a symptomatic criterion on a continuum).
NO = A dichotomous criterion statement is clearly **false.**
+   = **Threshold** (for a symptomatic criterion on a continuum).
YES = A dichotomous criterion statement is clearly **true.**

The majority of the SCID questions can be answered by a simple "YES" or "NO"; however, an unelaborated response of "YES" is rarely enough information to determine whether a criterion is met. Asking the patient to elaborate or provide specific examples is usually necessary to make a valid diagnostic rating. For instance, one of the questions for a Major Depressive Episode asks whether the patient has had "trouble thinking or concentrating." If the patient endorses this item as a problem, the clinician must ask follow-up probes before rating the criterion as "+" to ensure that the patient's experiences match the corresponding criterion (i.e., "Has it been hard to make decisions about everyday things? [What kinds of things has it been interfering with? Nearly every day?]"). A rating of "+" should be made only after the clinician is satisfied from the patient's responses that the criterion is met. Sometimes this entails rephrasing or paraphrasing the wording of the criterion to make the concept clearer to the patient. At other times, the clinician might find it necessary to seek corroborating information from other sources (e.g., family members, previous records).

Remember that it is not necessary for the patient to acknowledge that the symptom is present to justify a rating of "+" or not present to justify a rating of "—". (See Section 7.4, "Ratings of Criterion Items," in this User's Guide for more information about making ratings). The rating ultimately depends on the clinician making a clinical judgment as to whether or not a diagnostic criterion is met. If the clinician is confident that a particular symptom is present despite the patient's denial of the symptom, the clinician can gently challenge the response or even code the symptom as present ("+") if there is enough supporting evidence to do so (e.g., a patient who claims that spending 2 hours a day in a hand-washing ritual is not excessive or unreasonable). On the other hand, if the clinician doubts that a symptom is present even after hearing the patient describe it, the item should be rated as absent or subclinical ("—").

5.4   Diagnostic Summary Score Sheet

After the SCID-5-CV is completed, the clinician fills out the Diagnostic Summary Score Sheet (pages 1–6) indicating those DSM-5 diagnoses that were made during the interview. The Diagnostic Summary Score Sheet includes the corresponding ICD-10-CM diagnostic codes for each diagnosis. DSM-5 diagnoses are generally listed in the order that the diagnoses are made during the course of the SCID-5-CV evaluation. The clinician indicates the relevant DSM-5 diagnoses and coded subtype/specifiers and whether criteria are met currently or only in the past by checking the appropriate box on the SCID-5-CV Diagnostic Summary Score Sheet.

For those disorders preceded by two check boxes (e.g., Schizophrenia, Panic Disorder, PTSD), the left-hand box ("Current") should be checked if criteria have been currently met, and the right-hand box ("Past History") should be checked if criteria have been met only in the past. For the episodic mood disorders (i.e., Bipolar I Disorder, Bipolar II Disorder, Major Depressive Disorder), the left-hand box ("Current") should be checked for those severity specifiers that are present currently (i.e., Mild, Moderate, Severe, With Psychotic Features) and the right-hand box ("Past History") should be checked for those diagnoses In Partial Remission or In Full Remission. For those disorders preceded by a single box in the left-hand column (i.e., "Current" or "Past 12 Months"), the box should be checked if the criteria are currently met during the indicated time frame (e.g., the past 12 months). For those disorders (e.g., Psychotic Disorder Due to Another Medical Condition or Substance/Medication-Induced Depressive Disorder) preceded by a single box ("Lifetime") in the right-hand column, the box should be checked if the disorder has been present in the patient's lifetime. Note that because of the complexity of the diagnostic codes for the Substance/Medication-Induced Mental Disorders, which depend both on the class of substance and the severity of a comorbid Substance Use Disorder, the applicable diagnostic code must be written in by the clinician after consulting the appropriate coding table on page 6, as stated in the accompanying footnote. For example, in order to indicate a depressive disorder judged to be due to cocaine use in an individual with a Severe Cocaine Use Disorder, the clinician would check off the "Lifetime" box preceding Substance/Medication-Induced Depressive Disorder and indicate that the etiological substance was cocaine and the diagnostic code was F14.24 according to the coding table on page 6.

5.5 Sources of Information

The clinician should use all sources of information available about the patient in making the ratings. This might include referral notes and the observations of family members and friends. In some cases, the clinician may need to gently challenge a patient regarding discrepancies between his or her account and other sources of information.

If the patient is a poor historian (e.g., a hospitalized patient with acute psychotic symptoms and agitation, a chronic patient with cognitive impairment), much of the information may need to be drawn from the medical records or other sources. Before beginning to interview such a patient, the clinician should review the patient's medical records, note symptoms and dates of prior hospitalizations in the Treatment History Chart in the Overview section (on page 7), and record the pertinent symptoms in the appropriate section of the SCID-5-CV (e.g., record psychotic symptoms in Module B). In such cases, the SCID is not so much an interview guide as a place to systematically record symptoms that have been documented in the patient's records.

6. Administration of the SCID-5-CV

Ordinarily, the SCID-5-CV is administered in a single sitting and usually takes from 45 to 90 minutes, depending on the complexity of the psychiatric history and the ability of the patient to describe his or her psychopathology succinctly. Particularly complex cases can take up to 3 hours. In some cases, the SCID-5-CV may need to be administered over multiple sittings. If additional information becomes available after the interview is completed, the clinician should modify the SCID data accordingly.

Administration of the SCID by videoconferencing was compared with face-to-face assessment within a rural American Indian community in a study by Shore and colleagues (2007). The study found that SCID assessment by live interactive videoconferencing did not differ significantly from face-to-face assessment.

7. SCID-5-CV Conventions and Usage

Note: It is recommended that you have a copy of the SCID-5-CV in front of you while reviewing the next sections.

7.1 Item Labels

Each rated item in the SCID-5-CV has been assigned a label consisting of a capital letter (indicating the SCID-5-CV module) and a number. These item labels, which appear to the left and to the right of each item in the SCID-5-CV, serve several purposes.

- First and foremost, these item labels are used to control the diagnostic flow through the SCID-5-CV. All of the skip instructions in the SCID-5-CV use these item labels as target locations to inform the clinician of where to continue the interview. In the below example, which shows the questions and rating for Criterion A in current Hypomanic Episode (item label A41), if the clinician makes a rating of "—", he or she is instructed to skip to page 22 of the interview and continue with the assessment of past Manic Episode (beginning with item label A54).

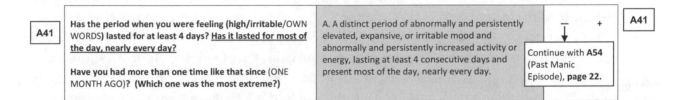

- Item labels are often used to reference item locations in the SCID-5-CV instructions for the clinician. For example, the instruction for assessing the Criterion B items in past Manic Episode informs the clinician that "FOR **A56–A62,** FOCUS ON THE MOST SEVERE PERIOD OF THE EPISODE THAT YOU ARE INQUIRING ABOUT." The referenced item labels A56–A62 correspond to the specific Manic Episode criteria in question.
- The ratings for a number of diagnostic criteria, especially those in Modules C and D, depend on the ratings of prior items. For example, Criterion A for Schizophrenia in Module C (two or more of the following: delusions, hallucinations…) depends on ratings of psychotic symptoms in Module B. Consequently, each component of Criterion A for Schizophrenia refers the clinician back to the relevant ratings made in Module B (e.g., "1. Delusions **[B1–B13]**, 2. Hallucinations **[B14–B19]**…").
- Finally, the item labels can be useful in situations in which the SCID-5-CV data are being entered into a computerized database. By adopting these item labels as variable names in the computer program, the SCID data can be more easily compared with other SCID databases that have been set up using this naming convention for the data fields.

7.2 Three-Column Format for Modules A, B, E, F, G, H, and J

In Modules A, B, E, F, G, H, and J, the left-hand column of each page consists of the SCID-5-CV interview questions (in bold) and directions (in capital letters) for the clinician. The DSM-5 diagnostic criteria to which the interview questions refer are in the middle column of the page. The right-hand column of each page contains the codes for rating the criteria. To the far left and far right, in small boxes, are the item labels described above in Section 7.1, "Item Labels."

7.3   SCID Questions

7.3.1   Questions asked verbatim

SCID questions not enclosed in parentheses are to be asked verbatim of every patient. The only exception to this basic SCID rule is in those instances in which the patient has already provided the necessary information earlier in the SCID-5-CV interview. For example, if during the Overview the patient states that the reason for coming to the clinic is that he or she has been very depressed for the past couple of months, the clinician would not then ask verbatim the initial question in Module A: "...has there been a period of time when you were feeling depressed or down most of the day, nearly every day?" In such instances, however, the clinician should NOT just assume that the symptom is present and code the item "+" without asking for confirmation, because some aspect of the criterion may not have been adequately explored (e.g., its duration or persistence for most of the day, nearly every day). Instead, the clinician should confirm the information already obtained by paraphrasing the original question. For example, the clinician may say "You've already told me that you were feeling depressed for the last couple of months. Was there a 2-week period in which you were depressed for most of the day, nearly every day?"

7.3.2   Questions enclosed in parentheses

The SCID convention is that questions in parentheses should be asked when necessary to clarify responses and can be skipped if the clinician already either knows the answer to the parenthetical question or has sufficient information to rate the criterion as "+". For example, the initial question for the "increase in goal-directed activity" item (Criterion B6, item label A36) in Manic Episode asks the patient how he or she has spent his or her time. If the patient provides a detailed recounting of behavior that clearly meets this criterion, there is no need to ask the additional parenthetical questions such as "Were you more sociable during that time, such as calling on friends, going out with them more than you usually do, or making a lot of new friends?" If, however, the patient's answer to the initial question is not sufficiently detailed to determine whether or not the criterion is met, the clinician should ask as many of the parenthetical questions as needed to be able to make that rating.

The fact that a question is in parentheses does not imply that the information the question is designed to elicit is any less critical. For instance, the first item (Criterion A1, item label A1) in Major Depressive Episode has the inquiry "As long as 2 weeks?" in parentheses. Unless the patient mentions the duration of the depressed mood, the clinician must ask if it lasted for as long as 2 weeks, because this duration of depressed mood is a critical requirement for rating this symptom as present.

7.3.3. "OWN WORDS" (and other phrases in all-capital letters, such as "AGORAPHOBIC SXS")

Many of the SCID questions contain phrases in all-capital letters enclosed in parentheses, such as "(OWN WORDS)," "(AGORAPHOBIC SXS)," and so forth. This convention indicates that the clinician is to modify the question and insert patient-specific words in place of these designations. For "OWN WORDS," the clinician should insert the words that the patient has been using to describe the particular symptom. For example, if the patient refers to a Manic Episode as "when I was wired," then the clinician might rephrase the question "When were you the most (high/irritable/OWN WORDS?)" to "When were you the most wired?" For phrases such as "(AGORAPHOBIC SXS)," the clinician should insert the particular symptoms that the patient has endorsed during the course of the interview. For example, the question corresponding to Criterion G (the clinical significance criterion; item label F29) for Agoraphobia asks "What effect have (AGORAPHOBIC SXS) had on your life?" In this circumstance, the clinician should insert the already acknowledged agoraphobic symptoms into the question (e.g., "What effect has your not being able to drive across bridges or go into crowded stores had on your life?").

7.3.4 "ONE MONTH AGO" (and other time intervals in all-capital letters)

Studies of memory and recall have demonstrated that individuals are more accurate in their recounting of events if questions are anchored to specific past dates as opposed to general time intervals. For this reason, questions inquiring about the presence of a symptom during a particular time interval (e.g., "During the past month") have been augmented or replaced by a phrase such as "since (ONE MONTH AGO)," requiring the clinician to use the exact date in the question. For example, in the determination of whether criteria for Manic Episode in Bipolar I Disorder are currently met (item label D17), the SCID question is "During the past month, since (ONE MONTH AGO), have you had (MANIC SXS RATED '+')?" For a SCID interview being done on December 15, the clinician would translate this into "During the past month, since the middle of November, have you had symptoms like not needing sleep, being very talkative, having a lot of energy, having racing thoughts, or being easily distracted?"

7.4 Ratings of Criterion Items

The majority of DSM-5 criteria require that a psychiatric sign, symptom, or finding be present at some sufficient level of severity, persistence, or duration in order to count toward the diagnosis. For such items, the SCID-5-CV offers two possible ratings: "—=absent/subthreshold" and "+=threshold." However, other criteria, such as those invoking diagnostic exclusion rules (e.g., "not better explained by another mental disorder"), as well as algorithmic statements (e.g., "AT LEAST THREE CRITERION A ITEMS ARE CODED "+"), have only two possible available ratings: "NO" and "YES." The SCID-5-CV ratings are explained as follows:

— = **Absent/Subthreshold:** The symptom described in the criterion is either clearly absent (e.g., no significant weight loss or weight gain or decrease or increase in appetite), or subthreshold (e.g., patient has been depressed for only 7 days rather than the required 2-week minimum; patient reports loss of interest in only a few activities, but not the required "almost all activities").

NO = The criterion statement is clearly **false** (e.g., for a criterion in the form of "the disturbance is not better explained by another mental disorder," code "NO" for situations in which the clinician decides that the disturbance is better explained by another mental disorder).

\+ = **Threshold:** The threshold for the criterion is just met (e.g., patient reports being depressed for 2 weeks) or more than met (e.g., patient reports being depressed for several months).

YES = The criterion statement is clearly **true** (e.g., at least three Criterion B symptoms are rated "+").

7.5   Note Format

The formatting of notes within the SCID-5-CV conveys particular meanings. "**Note**" in boldface reflects the inclusion of such notes as contained in the DSM-5 criteria. Other notes throughout the SCID-5-CV are italicized, with "*NOTE*" in all-capital letters; these notes indicate specific guidance or instructions for rating the criteria or conducting the SCID-5-CV interview.

7.6   Recording Descriptive Information

For most items, the clinician should ask the patient to provide specific details of thoughts, feelings, and behaviors to support the criterion ratings. This information should be recorded on the SCID in order to document the information used to justify the clinician's rating. For those criteria in which documentation of specific information is particularly important, the word "DESCRIBE" appears below the criterion. The clinician should clearly label information on the SCID that was obtained from sources other than the patient (e.g. charts, informant).

7.7   Skip Instructions

When moving through the SCID interview, the default rule is always to move to the next item unless otherwise instructed. This each-item-in-turn sequential flow is altered by skip instructions that facilitate skipping over diagnostic criteria that no longer need to be assessed (i.e., because the criteria for the disorder can no longer be met) or are no longer relevant (e.g., skipping the assessment of Persistent Depressive Disorder because criteria are already met for a Manic or Hypomanic Episode).

These skip instructions come in three basic formats:

1. **At the beginning of a section:** Many sections have instructions informing the clinician of conditions under which the entire section may be skipped. For example, the

assessment of Persistent Depressive Disorder in Module A, page 29, begins with the following instruction:

IF: THERE HAS EVER BEEN A MANIC OR HYPOMANIC EPISODE, SKIP THE ASSESSMENT OF PERSISTENT DEPRESSIVE DISORDER AND CONTINUE WITH **B1** (PSYCHOTIC SYMPTOMS), **PAGE 31**.

The clinician evaluates the conditional statement (i.e., whether there have been any Manic or Hypomanic Episodes) and, if true, continues the SCID-5-CV with item label B1, the first item in the assessment of Module B (Psychotic and Associated Symptoms).

2. **Under a set of ratings:** In these cases, a skip instruction is indicated in the right-hand column where the ratings are made, most typically in a text box hanging down from the rating of "—". This convention is used to enable the clinician to skip out of a diagnostic section when the criterion being evaluated is judged to be absent/subthreshold or false. The clinician should follow the vertical line down to the box containing the skip instruction, which tells the clinician to skip to the specified item label on the specified page, and continue the interview from that point onward.

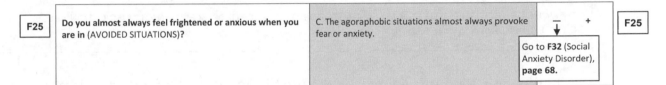

In the example above, taken from page 66 in the assessment of Agoraphobia, if a rating of "—" is given for Criterion C, the clinician should skip to item label **F32** on page 68 and resume asking questions from that point. Note that this does not indicate that the diagnosis is Social Anxiety Disorder but only directs the clinician to the assessment of Social Anxiety Disorder. If a rating of "+" is given, the clinician should proceed to the next item (i.e., item label F26, Criterion D in Agoraphobia), in keeping with the SCID rule that unless there is an instruction to the contrary, one should always continue with the next item.

In some cases, rather than having a text box (with a skip instruction) hanging from a rating of "—", there is an arrow leading to a box containing a follow-up question. This mechanism is often used in the assessment of episodic disorders (e.g., lifetime Major Depressive Episodes, Manic Episodes, Hypomanic Episodes) as a way of having the clinician consider whether there are episodes other than the one initially selected for evaluation that should be considered once the criteria are not met for the initially selected episode. For example, in the evaluation of past Major Depressive Episode (item label A25), if the clinician rates a "—" on the clinical significance criterion (indicating that the selected past episode did not cause clinically significant distress or impairment), the clinician should follow the arrow down from the "—" rating, which leads to the follow-up question about whether there were any other past episodes that caused even more distress or impairment.

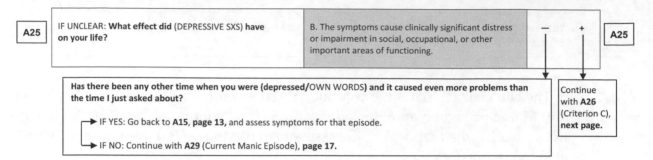

3. **As an instruction in the middle of the assessment of a disorder:** Skip instructions are sometimes indicated by capitalized instructions in the middle of a diagnostic assessment of a disorder. For example, at the conclusion of the drug history assessment (item labels E15a–E22a) on page 57, there is the following instruction:

> IF ANY CLASS OF ILLEGAL OR RECREATIONAL DRUGS WAS USED AT LEAST SIX TIMES WITHIN THE PAST 12 MONTHS OR PRESCRIBED/OTC MEDICATIONS WERE ABUSED OVER THE PAST 12 MONTHS (E.G., TAKING MORE THAN PRESCRIBED OR RECOMMENDED, DOCTOR SHOPPING TO GET PRESCRIPTIONS), GO TO **E23** (Past-12-Month Nonalcohol Substance Use Disorder), **page 58.**
>
> OTHERWISE (I.E., NO DRUG USED AT LEAST SIX TIMES AND NO EVIDENCE OF PRESCRIPTION/OTC MEDICATION ABUSE), GO TO **F1** (Panic Disorder), **page 63.**

In this case, the clinician reviews the use history for each of the drug classes and considers whether an illegal or recreational drug was used at least six times within the past 12 months or whether the patient abused any over-the-counter or prescribed medication. If not, the clinician is instructed to skip to the assessment of Panic Disorder, starting with item label F1 on page 63.

7.8   Decision Tree Format for Modules C and D

Module C (Differential Diagnosis of Psychotic Disorders) and Module D (Differential Diagnosis of Mood Disorders) use a decision tree format, in contrast to the other modules, which use the previously described three-column format. Each criterion is contained in a decision box, with two arrows, one labeled "YES" and the other labeled "NO," leading out from it. The clinician evaluates the criterion in the box based on symptom information obtained in Modules A and B. In some cases, additional information may be needed to evaluate the criteria, and additional clarifying interview questions are provided. If the criterion is present, the clinician rates the item "YES" by circling the word "YES" in the SCID-5-CV and follows the "YES" arrow to the next box; if the criterion is absent, the clinician rates the item "NO" by circling the word "NO" in the SCID-5-CV and follows the "NO" arrow to the next box.

The following example is from the assessment of Delusional Disorder and illustrates the assessment of Criterion B, item label C14, on page 40:

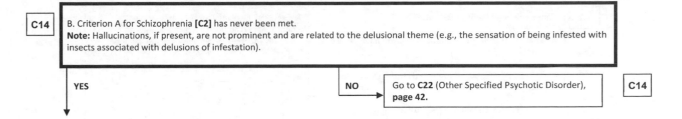

The clinician evaluates Criterion B after making a "YES" rating of Criterion A (item label C13). If Criterion B is true (i.e., Criterion A for Schizophrenia has never been met), the clinician circles the "YES" rating for item label C14 and continues with the evaluation of Criterion C in item label C15. If Criterion B is false (i.e., Criterion A for Schizophrenia has been met), the clinician circles the "NO" rating for item label C14 and continues with item label C22 (Other Specified Psychotic Disorder) on page 42.

7.9   Multiple Clauses in Criterion Sets

Many of the diagnostic criteria in DSM-5 contain multiple clauses that are joined by "OR" (e.g., there is a persistent desire OR unsuccessful efforts to cut down or control alcohol use). A rating of "+" for the criterion is made if ANY of the clauses are judged to be present. Typically there are multiple SCID interview questions for such criteria, with subsequent questions after the initial question preceded by "IF NO." Therefore, in order to maximize interviewing efficiency, the clinician only needs to ask the additional questions if the first part of the criterion is considered to be true. In the following example, if the patient answers "YES" to the first question and provides supporting examples, the item can be rated "+" without the clinician having to ask about whether the patient was drinking for a longer period of time than intended.

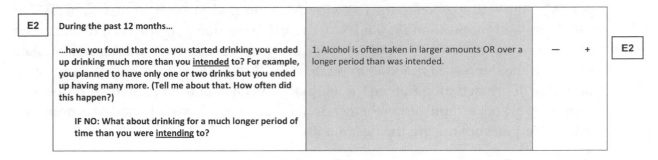

Note that for some criteria, particularly those in which each of the subcomponents of the criterion is of clinical importance (e.g., those in the Major Depressive Episode criteria set), the clinician must ask all of the questions corresponding to the components of the criterion regardless of whether the question corresponding to the initial part of the criterion is answered "YES" or "NO." For example, although Criterion A7 of Major Depressive Episode (item label A7) requires feelings of worthlessness OR excessive or inappropriate guilt, questions are provided to assess both of these components because of the clinical importance of both of these symptoms.

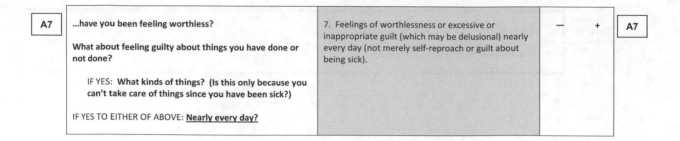

7.10   Brackets Indicating Mutually Exclusive Questions

Pairs of mutually exclusive questions are indicated by a bracket connecting the pair of questions on the left-hand side of the page. In such situations, the clinician decides which of the pair of questions should be read next by examining the capitalized conditional statements to see which of the two questions applies. For example, in the assessment of current Major Depressive Episode (item label A2, page 10), the question for the loss of interest item (Criterion A2) begins with the following pair of mutually exclusive questions:

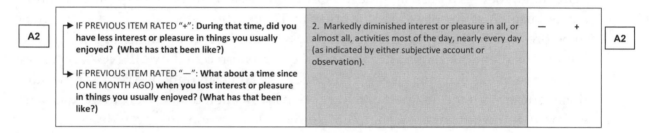

In this case, the selection of the particular version of the loss of interest question depends on the rating given to the Criterion A1 depressed mood item (item label A1). If the depressed mood item is rated "+", the first selection is made (i.e., determining whether or not there was loss of interest during the time of the 2 weeks of depressed mood). If the depressed mood item is rated "—" (indicating that there was no 2-week period of depressed mood), then the alternative version of the loss of interest question should be asked, establishing whether or not there was a 2-week period of diminished interest or pleasure during the past month.

7.11   Due to General Medical Condition, Substance/ Medication-Induced, or Primary

Most of the diagnoses covered in the SCID-5-CV include a criterion that requires the clinician to decide whether or not the psychopathology is caused by the direct effects of a general medical condition (GMC) or substance/medication use on the central nervous system (e.g., "the disturbance is not attributable to the physiological effects of a substance [e.g., a drug of abuse, a medication] or another medical condition"). If the clinician determines that the disturbance is not due to the direct physiological effects of a GMC or substance/medication use, the symptoms are considered to be **primary,** and the clinician continues to the next item (which most typically results in making the diagnosis because the "organic rule-out" criterion is usually the last item in the criteria set). If, instead, the clinician judges that the symptoms are in fact due to the direct effects of a GMC or substance/medication use, then the clinician is instructed to skip out of the evaluation and instead diagnose the appropriate Mental Disorder Due to Another Medical Condition or Substance/Medication-Induced Mental Disorder and to indicate the corresponding disorder (and ICD-10-CM diagnostic code) on the Diagnostic Summary Score Sheet. (See Section 9, "Differentiating General Medical and Substance/Medication Etiologies From Primary Disorders," for guidelines about how the clinician should make this determination.)

For example, in evaluating the criteria for a Major Depressive Episode, the clinician comes to item label A12, Criterion C ("not attributable to the physiological effects of a substance [e.g., a drug of abuse, a medication] or another medical condition"). If the clinician decides that the depression is secondary to cocaine use occurring in the context of a Severe Cocaine Use Disorder, then a diagnosis of Substance/Medication-Induced Depressive Disorder is made, the "Lifetime" box is checked off in front of Substance/Medication-Induced Depressive Disorder on the Diagnostic Summary Score Sheet, and the clinician would indicate that the specific substance is cocaine and that the diagnostic code is F14.24. On the other hand, if the clinician decides that the depression is primary (or independent of the substance/medication or the GMC), the clinician continues with item label A13, on the next page (i.e., "Onset of depression (month/year)").

NEOPHYTE SCIDers BEWARE: The double negative in this criterion is a common source of confusion. The exclusion criterion **IS MET** (rated "YES") if the disturbance is **NOT** due to a substance/medication or GMC (i.e., it is primary)—say to yourself, "YES, there is no substance/medication or GMC that is causing the psychiatric symptoms (or, to recall that chestnut from the 1920s, "Yes, we have no bananas!"). The criterion is **NOT MET** (rated "NO") if it is **NOT TRUE** that the disturbance is not due to a substance/medication or GMC—say to yourself "NO, there is a substance/medication or a GMC that is causing the psychiatric symptoms."

Note that throughout the SCID-5, the DSM-IV term *general medical condition* has been retained to refer to nonpsychiatric medical conditions instead of the DSM-5 term *another medical condition*. The GMC term was chosen to prevent any confusion arising from the fact that "another medical condition" could be interpreted to include psychiatric conditions as well as medical conditions. A psychiatric disorder is in fact "another medical condition" as per the DSM-5 perspective that considers all psychiatric disorders to be medical conditions. The term *another medical condition* is used in the SCID-5 only when referring to the name of a DSM-5 disorder (e.g., Depressive Disorder Due to Another Medical Condition) or when it appears within a DSM-5 diagnostic criterion (e.g., "the episode is not attributable to the physiological effects of a substance (e.g., a drug of abuse, a medication) or another medical condition)." More specific instructions for determining whether a disturbance is due to a GMC, is substance/medication-induced, or is primary are found in Section 9, "Differentiating General Medical and Substance/Medication Etiologies From Primary Disorders."

7.12   Consideration of Treatment Effects

Symptoms should be coded as present or absent <u>without</u> any assumptions about what would have been present if the patient were not receiving treatment. Thus, if a patient with Schizophrenia is taking 12 mg/day of risperidone and is no longer delusional or hearing voices, psychotic symptoms are considered to be currently absent for the purposes of determining whether the diagnosis of Schizophrenia is "current," even if the clinician believes that without the medication the hallucinations would probably have been present. Similarly, if a patient is taking a hypnotic medication every night and no longer has problems sleeping, insomnia should be coded as currently absent ("—") in the assessment of current Major Depressive Episode.

7.13   Clinical Significance

Most disorders in the SCID-5 include a criterion that requires there to be clinically significant distress or impairment before a DSM-5 diagnosis can be made. Note that there are two components, distress and impairment, either of which indicates clinical significance. It is usually more straightforward to determine what constitutes clinically significant impairment rather than clinically significant distress; therefore, the SCID-5 impairment questions come first. Thus, distress only needs to be assessed in those relatively uncommon circumstances in which there is distress without any impairment. (It is often helpful to think of the "distress" component in terms of how much the patient is bothered by the fact that he or she has the symptoms.) The initial question asks about how the symptoms have affected the patient's life. Usually the answer to that question is enough to determine the clinical significance of the symptoms. However, if the impact on the patient's life remains unclear, there are a number of optional questions included to assess the impact of the symptoms on work and school functioning, social functioning, leisure activities, and other areas of functioning. DSM-5 does not provide any guidelines as to how much impairment is needed to be considered "clinically significant"—leaving it to the judgment of the clinician. Certainly, seeking treatment is evidence of clinically significant distress or impairment, but even that rule of thumb may not be helpful in determining whether comorbid symptoms that are uncovered during the evaluation process should be considered clinically significant.

7.14   Other Specified and Unspecified Disorders

DSM-5 replaced the DSM-IV Not Otherwise Specified (NOS) designation with two options for clinical use: Other Specified Disorder and Unspecified Disorder. According to DSM-5 (pp. 15–16)—

> The other specified disorder category is provided to allow the clinician to communicate the specific reason that the presentation does not meet the criteria for any specific category within a diagnostic class. This is done by recording the name of the category, followed by the specific reason. For example, for an individual with clinically significant depressive symptoms lasting 4 weeks but whose symptomatology falls short of the diagnostic threshold for a major depressive episode, the clinician would record "other

specified depressive disorder, depressive episode with insufficient symptoms." If the clinician chooses not to specify the reason that the criteria are not met for a specific disorder, then "unspecified depressive disorder" would be diagnosed.

The SCID-5-CV includes three Other Specified/Unspecified categories: Other Specified/Unspecified Schizophrenia Spectrum and Other Psychotic Disorder, Other Specified/Unspecified Bipolar and Related Disorder, and Other Specified/Unspecified Depressive Disorder. As in DSM-5, the Other Specified/Unspecified categories are to be diagnosed for presentations in which symptoms characteristic of a Schizophrenia Spectrum and Other Psychotic Disorder, Bipolar and Related Disorder, or Depressive Disorder predominate but do not meet the full criteria for any of the disorders in the respective diagnostic class.

Note that throughout the SCID-5-CV interview, the DSM-5 Other Specified Disorder and Unspecified Disorder categories are combined into a single category: Other Specified Disorder. The difference depends entirely on coding and recording issues (i.e., "Other Specified" applies if the clinician chooses to indicate the reason why the presentation did not meet criteria for a specific disorder in the diagnostic class, and "Unspecified" applies if the clinician chooses *not* to indicate the reason). The clinician will differentiate between the "Other Specified" and "Unspecified" categories only on the Diagnostic Summary Score Sheet, which also includes the corresponding diagnostic code for each diagnosis. Thus, if the clinician records the presence of Other Specified Disorder on the Diagnostic Summary Score Sheet, the clinician is expected to write in the reason that the criteria for a specific disorder are not met. Space is provided on the Diagnostic Summary Score Sheet to provide the reason.

As noted on the Diagnostic Summary Score Sheet, a coding exception applies to Other Specified Bipolar Disorder. Presentations that meet criteria for Cyclothymic Disorder (which is included in the SCID-5-RV but not the SCID-5-CV) are to be assigned the diagnostic code F34.0 for Cyclothymic Disorder instead of F31.89, the diagnostic code for Other Specified Bipolar Disorder.

7.15   Deviations From DSM-5 Criteria

The middle column in the SCID-5-CV generally contains the DSM-5 criteria reprinted verbatim. There are several circumstances in which the diagnostic criteria deviate from the verbatim DSM-5. In the course of revising the SCID, we discovered several apparent errors and ambiguities in the DSM-5 criteria and inconsistencies between the DSM-5 criteria and the accompanying explanatory text. In such situations, after consulting with members of the DSM-5 Work Groups in order to confirm that these were in fact errors and to arrive at the best solution, we made changes in the DSM-5 criteria sets to reflect the outcome of these discussions. In other cases, changes have been made to enhance the SCID interview. For example, the illustrative examples that accompanied the DSM-IV criteria for Substance Dependence and Substance Abuse that were omitted from DSM-5 have been included in the SCID. An explanation of these adjustments to the DSM-5 criteria wording and the rationale for our corrections is included in the annotations of the individual criteria in Section 10, "Special Instructions for Individual Modules."

Whenever the DSM-5 criteria in the SCID differ from what is in the official DSM-5, we have noted the changes by bracketing the text:

- Phrases <u>added</u> to the DSM-5 diagnostic criteria are enclosed in brackets (e.g., item label F41, Criterion J in Social Anxiety Disorder: "If another medical condition (e.g., Parkinson's disease, obesity, disfigurement from burns or injury) [or potentially embarrassing mental disorder] is present, the fear, anxiety, or avoidance is clearly unrelated or is excessive."
- Words that have been <u>omitted</u> are indicated with a bracketed ellipse (e.g., item label D3, Criterion B for Bipolar I Disorder, in which the words "or Unspecified Schizophrenia Spectrum and Other" are omitted, per discussion in Section 7.14, "Other Specified and Unspecified Disorders": "The occurrence of the Manic and Major Depressive Episode(s) is not better explained by Schizoaffective Disorder, Schizophrenia, Schizophreniform Disorder, Delusional Disorder, or Other Specified [...] Psychotic Disorder").

For editorial reasons, we retained the DSM-IV convention of capitalizing disorder and specifier names so as to more clearly set these diagnostic constructs off from the rest of the text. For similar reasons, we also decided to retain the DSM-IV term "general medical condition" (GMC) throughout the SCID-5 instructions to refer to medical conditions listed outside of the mental disorders chapter in the *International Classification of Diseases* (ICD), rather than use the DSM-5 term "another medical condition." However, we did retain the use of "another medical condition" (or "AMC") when it appears within a DSM-5 diagnostic criterion and when it occurs as part of the name of the disorder (e.g., the SCID-5-CV Diagnostic Summary Score Sheet refers to "Depressive Disorder Due to Another Medical Condition").

8.   SCID Do's and Don'ts

DO	DON'T
DO give the patient a brief explanation of the purpose of the interview before beginning.	**DON'T** apologize for the questions you are asking or the length of the interview. Most patients appreciate the thoroughness of the SCID and welcome the opportunity to describe their symptoms in detail.
DO use the Overview to establish rapport and set the tone for the interview. Be present with the patient, demonstrating a nonjudgmental stance while showing appropriate professionalism and boundaries.	**DON'T** let challenging patients take control of the interview: • **DON'T** let patients be unnecessarily tangential. Redirect patients who are providing information that is unnecessary for completing a diagnostic interview. • **DON'T** be defensive with patients who are angry or hostile. Use reflective statements to demonstrate empathy. **DON'T** ignore a patient's reports of suffering. Demonstrate empathy while maintaining an objective stance.
DO use the Overview to collect information about the patient's symptoms and functioning to inform the questions you'll ask in the diagnostic modules.	**DON'T** ask detailed questions in the Overview about specific symptoms that are covered in the later sections of the SCID.
DO get enough of an Overview of the current illness at the beginning of the interview to understand the context in which the illness developed.	**DON'T** ask the specific questions about symptoms after a perfunctory overview of a current illness.
DO use open-ended questions to capture the patient's perceptions of the problem in his or her own words.	**DON'T** ask leading questions. Keep an open mind about hypotheses. Use closed-ended questions sparingly.
DO stick to the initial questions, as they are written, except for necessary minor modifications to take into account what the patient has already said.	**DON'T** make up your own initial questions because you think you have a better way of getting at the same information. Your minor improvement may have a major unwanted effect on the meaning of the question. Great care was taken in crafting the exact phrasing of each question, and the questions work in nearly all cases.
DO ask additional clarifying questions in order to elicit details in the patient's own words, such as "Can you tell me about that?" or "Do you mean that…?"	**DON'T** use the interview as a checklist or true/false test.

DO	DON'T
DO pay attention to consistency in patients' reports and what is known about the symptoms. **DO** gently challenge discrepancies.	**DON'T** be afraid of offending the patient by asking more follow-up questions. In fact, when you seek to clarify responses, patients may be more likely to feel that they are being truly heard.
DO make sure that you and the patient are focusing on the same (and the appropriate) time period for each question.	**DON'T** assume that symptoms cluster together in time unless you have clarified the time period. For example, the patient may be talking about a symptom that occurred a year ago and another symptom that appeared last week, when you are focusing on symptoms that occurred jointly during a 2-week period of possible Major Depressive Episode.
DO focus on obtaining the information necessary to judge all of the requirements of a criterion under consideration. As noted above, this may require asking additional questions.	**DON'T** focus only on getting a "YES" or "NO" answer to the SCID question.
DO give the patient the benefit of any doubt about a questionable psychotic symptom by rating "—".	**DON'T** call a subculturally accepted religious belief or an overvalued idea a delusion. **DON'T** confuse ruminations or obsessions with auditory hallucinations.
DO make sure that each symptom noted as present is diagnostically significant.	**DON'T** assume that a symptom is diagnostically significant just because it is endorsed. For example, if a patient says that "YES," he had trouble sleeping, but he has always had trouble sleeping, then that symptom should not be noted as present in the portion of the SCID dealing with the diagnosis of a Major Depressive Episode unless the sleep problem was worse during the period under review. This is particularly important when an episodic condition (such as a Major Depressive Episode) is superimposed on a chronic condition (such as Persistent Depressive Disorder).
DO pay attention to double negatives, especially in the exclusion criteria. Remember to use the phrase "Yes, we have no bananas" to help guide you if you get confused about how you should rate one of these criteria. For example, if the patient denies using drugs or medications or being ill during the onset of a disturbance, "YES," it is true that no medical condition or substance use is causing the disturbance.	**DON'T** code "NO" for an exclusion criterion requiring the <u>absence</u> of etiological factors when what you mean to indicate is that the excluded etiological factors are *not* present (and thus the criterion should be rated "YES"). For example, if the criterion reads "not attributable to the physiological effects of a substance or another medical condition," then a rating of "NO" means that the disturbance is secondary (i.e., due to a GMC or substance/medication), and a rating of "YES" means that the disturbance is primary—NOT due to a GMC or substance/medication.

9.   Differentiating General Medical and Substance/ Medication Etiologies From Primary Disorders

This section describes the process of evaluating the organic rule-out criterion that is included in the diagnostic criteria for the majority of the disorders assessed in the SCID, usually as one of the last items in each diagnostic criteria set. This criterion occurs typically in the following form: "The disturbance is not attributable to the physiological effects of a substance (e.g., a drug of abuse, a medication) or another medical condition." The first consideration when evaluating this criterion is whether, **at the time of onset or worsening of the symptoms,** the patient was physically ill with a GMC (either acute or chronic), taking a medication, or using significant amounts of alcohol or a drug of abuse. Consequently, the SCID-5-CV questions that correspond to this criterion begin with the following: "Just before this began, were you physically ill?" "Just before this began, were you taking any medications?" and "Just before this began, were you drinking or using any street drugs?" If there is no medical illness, medication use, or substance use coincident with the onset or worsening of the symptoms (i.e., the answers to these three questions are "NO"), then this criterion is automatically fulfilled and the clinician can give a "YES" rating for the item, indicating that the disturbance is primary. It is important to understand that the time frame of inquiry is NOT necessarily the artificially restricted period of time being focused on in the diagnostic assessment (e.g., worst 2 weeks in the past month for a potential current Major Depressive Episode or worst week of a potential past Manic Episode), but rather the point in time when the symptoms began or significantly worsened. It is therefore crucial at this point in the SCID-5-CV to know when the symptomatic period began. For that reason, the three questions noted above are preceded by a question such as: "If UNKNOWN: When did this period of (SYMPTOMS) begin?"

The next consideration is whether or not the medical illness, medication, or drug of abuse has the potential to cause the symptoms in question. To assist the clinician in making this determination, a list of symptom-specific etiological GMCs and etiological substances/medications, which were adapted for the most part from the DSM-5 text, are included with the criterion.[1]

The following two sections discuss the issues that need to be considered when determining whether the psychiatric symptoms are caused by the direct effects of the GMC or substance/medication use on the central nervous system. If the clinician concludes that the symptoms are in fact caused by either a GMC or substance/medication, the appropriate diagnosis (i.e., Mental Disorder Due to Another Medical Condition or Substance/Medication-Induced Mental Disorder) is indicated in the section of the SCID-5-CV Diagnostic Summary Score Sheet. For example, consider the evaluation of a patient with recurrent unexpected panic attacks. Criterion C for Panic Disorder (item label F20)

---

[1] The DSM-5 text for Bipolar and Related Disorders did not provide such a list, and we would like to thank Ariel Gildengers, M.D., and Antoine Doualhy, M.D., at the University of Pittsburgh Medical Center for their assistance with this list.

asks the clinician to consider whether the panic attacks are attributable to physiological effects of a substance or a GMC. If the patient were to acknowledge that he or she drinks five cups of coffee a day, the clinician should consider the possibility that the panic attacks are etiologically related to the heavy caffeine intake and inquire of the patient about the temporal relationship between the caffeine intake and the panic attacks. If the clinician were to then discover that the panic attacks occur only during periods of heavy coffee use, then the clinician would rate "NO" for this criterion (i.e., it is NOT true that the symptoms are NOT attributable to the physiological effects of a substance), the clinician would make a diagnosis of Caffeine-Induced Anxiety Disorder, and then skip to F23 (Agoraphobia), as instructed. Then at the conclusion of the interview, the clinician would indicate the presence of Caffeine-Induced Anxiety Disorder by placing a check in the "Lifetime" box preceding Substance/Medication-Induced Anxiety Disorder, and write in both the substance (i.e., "caffeine") and the ICD-10-CM diagnostic code (F15.980).

9.1   Guidelines for Determining Whether Symptoms Are Due to a General Medical Condition

This section offers guidelines for helping the clinician to evaluate the "due to a general medical condition" component of the organic rule-out criterion, which is based on the DSM-5 diagnostic criteria for Mental Disorders Due to Another Medical Condition. Once the presence of a GMC that has the potential to cause the psychiatric symptoms is established, the next step is to determine whether there is a close temporal relationship between the course of the psychiatric symptoms and the course of the GMC. For example, did the psychiatric symptoms start after the onset of the GMC, get better or get worse with the waxing and waning of the GMC, and remit when the GMC resolved?

Note that demonstrating a close temporal relationship does not necessarily imply that the causality is on a physiological level, which is an essential feature of a Mental Disorder Due to Another Medical Condition. A psychological reaction to the medical condition, as would be the case with the diagnosis of an Adjustment Disorder, would likely be characterized by a close temporal relationship as well. For example, depression occurring immediately after a paralyzing stroke could reflect damage to underlying brain structures responsible for regulating mood (causality at a physiological level) or may be a psychological reaction to the devastating loss of the ability to move a part of the body (causality at a psychological level). Furthermore, the lack of a temporal relationship does not necessarily rule out causality. In some instances, psychiatric symptoms may be the first harbinger of a GMC and may precede by months or years any physical manifestations (e.g., hypothyroidism, low testosterone, brain tumor). Conversely, psychiatric symptoms may be a relatively late manifestation, occurring months or years following the onset of a GMC (e.g., depression in Parkinson's disease).

Another factor that may suggest an etiological relationship between the GMC and the psychiatric symptoms is atypicality in symptom presentation. For example, severe weight loss in the face of a relatively mild depression, or the first onset of mania in an elderly patient, are unusual presentations and should alert the clinician to the possibility that a comorbid GMC is the cause. It should be acknowledged, however, that atypicality is not necessarily compelling evidence because, by their very nature, psychiatric presentations are quite heterogeneous within a particular diagnosis.

Finally, it is important for the clinician to consider whether a primary or Substance/Medication-Induced Mental Disorder best explains the symptoms. Are the psychiatric symptoms best explained as a psychological reaction to the stressor of having the GMC (in which case the diagnosis of Adjustment Disorder would be more appropriate)? Has the patient had prior episodes of the same type of psychiatric symptoms that were not due to a GMC (e.g., past recurrent depressive episodes)? Is the person abusing a substance or taking a medication that is known to cause the psychiatric symptoms? Does the patient have a strong family history for the disorder in question?

Note that the diagnoses that are "…Due to Another Medical Condition" are relatively rare. Much more common are the situations in which psychiatric symptoms are comorbid with a GMC (e.g., depression and heart disease). Therefore, when in doubt, the clinician's default position should be to assume that a GMC is NOT etiological (i.e., the psychiatric disorder is primary).

9.2   Assessing Substance/Medication-Induced Mental Disorders

This section offers guidelines for helping the clinician to evaluate the "due to the physiological effects of a substance" component of the organic rule-out criterion. In DSM-5, the term "substance/medication use" includes the use of illicit drugs and prescribed or over-the-counter medication. When substance/medication use and psychiatric symptoms co-occur, there are three possibilities as to the nature of their relationship to each other:

1. The psychiatric symptoms may be a direct physiological consequence of the substance/medication use (e.g., Cocaine-Induced Depressive Disorder, With Onset During Withdrawal).
2. The substance/medication use may be a manifestation of the psychiatric disorder (e.g., cocaine use to self-medicate an underlying depressive disorder).
3. The psychiatric symptoms and the substance/medication use may be coincidental.

A diagnosis of a Substance/Medication-Induced Mental Disorder is made in cases in which the first type of causal connection applies. Otherwise, a diagnosis of a primary psychiatric disorder is made.

In order to make the diagnosis of a Substance/Medication-Induced Mental Disorder, it must first be established that there is a temporal relationship between substance/medication use and the development of the psychiatric symptoms, and that the substance/medication use, at the dose and duration used by the patient, is sufficient to credibly cause the psychiatric symptoms. Furthermore, the clinician also needs to take into account other non-substance-related explanations for the symptoms before concluding that they are substance-induced (e.g., that the symptoms represent a recurrence of a long-standing mental disorder).

The following three guidelines for determining whether there is evidence that the symptoms are NOT substance/medication-induced are based on Criteria B and C in "Substance/Medication-Induced Mental Disorders" in DSM-5 (p. 488). If any of the three are true, then it can reasonably be concluded that the symptoms are NOT due to the direct physiological effects of a substance or medication, and thus the symptoms would be considered to be "primary."

1. **Is there evidence that the psychiatric symptoms preceded the onset of the substance/medication use?** A definite history of the psychiatric symptoms occurring before the course of substance/medication use suggests the second of the three causal scenarios (i.e., self-medication) and strongly supports the hypothesis that the symptoms cannot be explained by substance/medication use.

2. **Do the psychiatric symptoms persist, even after a substantial period of abstinence (e.g., about 1 month)?** If the symptoms were caused by the substance/medication use, then it is expected that they would remit after the acute effects of intoxication and withdrawal subside. If the symptoms continue to persist long after the substance/medication use ends, it suggests instead that the symptoms represent a primary mental disorder (or perhaps a Mental Disorder Due to Another Medical Condition). Although DSM-5 suggests that waiting 1 month after substance/medication use ends is sufficient, this 1-month waiting period should be considered only as a loose guideline. The actual amount of time of abstinence that would be required before concluding that the psychiatric symptoms are primary depends on many factors, including the particular substance/medication used, dosage, and half-life.

3. **Is there any other evidence that is more supportive of a primary psychiatric disorder or of a disorder due to a GMC accounting for the psychiatric symptoms?** The clinician should take into account such factors as a strong family history for the primary psychiatric disorder, prior episodes of these psychiatric symptoms that were unrelated to substance/medication use, and evidence for an etiological GMC.

10.   Special Instructions for Individual Modules

The next sections of the User's Guide provide specific instructions for each of the individual SCID modules. It is recommended that you have a copy of the SCID-5-CV to refer to while reviewing these sections.

10.1   SCID-5-CV Diagnostic Summary Score Sheet

The SCID-5-CV Diagnostic Summary Score Sheet provides a summary of those DSM-5 diagnoses (with their diagnostic codes) that were determined to be currently present or present in the past. The item label and page reference listed after each diagnosis indicate where in the SCID-5-CV that diagnosis was made and the location that the clinician should refer to in order to determine whether or not the diagnosis is current. For example, the item label C25 and the page number 44 follow the diagnosis of Schizophrenia in the Diagnostic Summary Score Sheet. On page 44, the first item (labeled C25) is where the diagnosis of Schizophrenia was made. If item C25 was rated as being "Current," the clinician should check the box under the "Current" column in front of the diagnosis of Schizophrenia in the Diagnostic Summary Score Sheet. If it is not rated as being current but instead was diagnosed as "Past Hx," the clinician should check the box in the "Past History" column in the Diagnostic Summary Score Sheet. Many diagnoses in the SCID-5-CV are only assessed for the current time period. In such cases, there is only one box in front of the diagnosis; it should be checked if the diagnosis is currently present.

The Mental Disorders Due to Another Medical Condition and Substance/Medication-Induced Mental Disorders, which may be diagnosed in the course of ruling out a GMC or substance/medication as the etiology for a disturbance, can only be diagnosed as "Lifetime" in the Diagnostic Summary Score Sheet. These disorders have multiple page references (with corresponding item labels) following the diagnosis in the Diagnostic Summary Score Sheet (e.g., Bipolar and Related Disorder Due to Another Medical Condition: p. 19/**A40,** p. 22/**A53**, p. 25/**A65**, p. 28/**A77,** p. 47/**D10**) because they are diagnosed in multiple locations in the SCID-5-CV (e.g., in the context of the evaluation of those criteria within Current Manic Episode, Current Hypomanic Episode, Past Manic Episode, and Past Hypomanic Episode, and Other Specified Bipolar Disorder that rule out a GMC or substance/medication-induced etiology).

10.2   Overview

The introductory Overview section is the foundation of the SCID-5-CV and serves a number of important functions:

1. Establishing rapport between the clinician and patient before delving into the patient's psychopathology.
2. Allowing the patient to describe his or her psychopathology in his or her own words.
3. Providing a contextual basis for the development of symptoms.
4. Determining the patient's current functioning, which may be useful for determining the clinical significance of current symptoms.
5. Exploring the patient's past functioning, which may be useful for determining the time of onset of disorders, the presence of undiagnosed psychiatric conditions, and possible comorbid medical conditions and substance/medication use, some of which may have a role in the etiology of current or past psychopathology.
6. Determining current and past suicidal ideation and attempts.
7. Revealing the presence of a current or past delusional belief system in a patient who does not have insight into his or her psychosis.

Sometimes the only indication of the presence of delusions is the patient's report during the Overview of behavior or thinking that is unusual or atypical and does not make immediate sense to the clinician, such as a patient with a persecutory delusion who reports that he or she has filed several lawsuits against the U.S. Postal Service for mail tampering.

Given that the questions included in the Overview potentially cover the patient's entire life history, the challenge in doing the Overview is getting sufficient information to understand the "landscape" of the patient's life history (i.e., the rough sequence of psychiatric events) without getting caught up in details. Moreover, the clinician should not go into detail about the patient's symptoms during the Overview because these will be extensively covered inside the individual SCID modules; the one exception is psychotic symptoms, which should be explored in detail at the point they arise during the Overview. For example, if the patient reports that he came for treatment because he was hearing voices, the clinician should immediately follow up by inquiring about the specific details concerning the voices (e.g., "How many voices? What were they saying to you?") and NOT wait until the psychotic symptom evaluation in Module B to inquire about the specifics of the voices.

The Overview generally takes approximately 15–30 minutes, although patients with particularly complex histories or who are poor historians can take considerably longer. Clinicians going through the Overview should be aware of common errors that may be made in either of two ways: 1) not following up on important pieces of information provided by the patient (e.g., not inquiring about the details and context of a past hospitalization for a suicide attempt), or 2) going into excessive detail about information that may be relevant for treatment planning but is not relevant to making a SCID diagnosis (e.g., obtaining the names and exact dosages of every medication that the patient has taken during his or her lifetime).

The Overview consists almost entirely of open-ended questions that mirror a general clinical interview. Thus, unlike the other sections of the SCID in which the clinician is expected to adhere closely to both the wording of the questions as well as their sequence, the clinician is allowed much greater flexibility in terms of changing both the sequence and wording of the questions if it makes clinical sense to do so, as long as all of the information covered in the Overview is eventually collected. For example, if at the beginning of the interview, in response to the question "With whom do you live?" the patient explains that he just started living in a halfway house after his recent hospitalization for hallucinations that commanded him to burn down his parent's house, it would make sense to immediately inquire about the circumstances of his recent hospitalization, as well as obtain more details about his recent psychotic symptoms rather than just continuing with the next question in the Overview ("What kind of work do you do?").

The initial questions serve mostly to establish rapport as well as to provide some contextual information that might be a clue to possible psychopathology (e.g., the fact that the person is living in a halfway house suggests current or past history of a relatively severe psychiatric condition). The questions about work history are often helpful in detecting a current or past history of psychopathology. For example, a history of interrupted schooling, problematic work history, being on disability, and so forth, are all potential clues to psychopathology and demand careful follow-up to determine the reasons for these problems.

The next sections focus on the presence of current psychopathology, treatment history, and medical history. The clinician should be sure to question the patient about any medications that were prescribed that do not seem appropriate for the condition described. This often gives a clue to problems that the patient has not mentioned. For example, a patient who describes only chronic depression, but was treated with lithium in the past, may describe a possible Manic Episode when asked why lithium was prescribed. Of course, neither a prescribed medication nor a previous diagnosis should be used to justify making a SCID-5-CV diagnosis without documentation that the disorder actually met criteria. When asking about a history of past treatment and it becomes clear that the patient has had a particularly complicated history, it may be useful to turn to the Treatment History chart, located about midway on the Overview page (and continued on page 9). This chart provides a framework for recording past treatment history in a chronological fashion.

When the SCID-5-CV is used to interview patients with psychotic symptoms who have limited insight into their illness, it is often necessary to rely on ancillary information to elicit responses in the Overview. For example, if a patient has no chief complaint and denies having any idea of why he or she was brought to a psychiatric unit, the clinician might say the following: "The admission note said you were burning your clothes in the bathtub, and your mother called the police. What was that all about?" In many cases in which the patient is currently psychotic, most of the information may need to come from the chart or from other informants.

The next section of the Overview assesses suicidal ideation and behavior, both lifetime and in the past week. In prior editions of the SCID, suicidality was only assessed in the context of evaluating Criterion A9 in current or past Major Depressive Episode. Because suicidal ideation and behavior may be associated with a wide variety of disorders besides Major Depressive Disorder, questions have been added to the Overview to assess suicidality both for diagnostic reasons (e.g., to identify particularly severe past periods of psychopathology) and for the purpose of assessing current patient safety.

The Overview then focuses on the current time period ("Other Current Problems") and inquires about potential stressors, current mood, and current alcohol and drug use.

10.3   Module A.   Evaluation of Mood Episodes and Persistent Depressive Disorder

Module A assesses current and past Major Depressive, Manic, and Hypomanic Episodes, and Persistent Depressive Disorder. The actual diagnoses of Bipolar I Disorder, Bipolar II Disorder, and Major Depressive Disorder are made in Module D using information collected in Module A, as well as the results of the evaluation of psychotic symptoms and psychotic disorders in Modules B and C, respectively.

10.3.1   Ratings for Current Major Depressive Episode (A1–A14)

Criterion A.   *Establishing the minimum 2-week duration.*   When the clinician begins to ask about a possible Major Depressive Episode (MDE), the first task is to determine whether there has been a 2-week period of depressed mood and/or diminished interest or pleasure that has occurred in the last month. If there is some doubt about whether the duration of the depressed mood has truly been 2 full weeks, the clinician should inquire about the specific symptoms anyway, because it often turns out that a patient who minimizes a problem when first asked, may on further reflection recall that he or she was, in fact, symptomatic for a full 2 weeks.

Establishing co-occurrence of symptoms during the same 2-week period.   Once it has been determined that depressed mood or diminished interest or pleasure has persisted most of the day, nearly every day, for at least 2 weeks, the next task is to determine whether at least four additional symptoms have occurred nearly every day during the same 2-week period. This is done by first establishing with the patient a "target" 2-week period within the past month and then making sure that the patient is aware that the next questions refer only to this 2-week period by periodically reminding the patient of the time frame when asking the questions (e.g., "during the first 2 weeks of the past month, how have you been sleeping?"). Any 2-week period in the past month can serve as the target—it is generally recommended that the clinician focus on what the patient perceives as the worst 2 weeks in the past month. If the patient reports that the depressed mood has been pretty much the same for the entire month, the clinician should focus on the most recent 2 weeks. Note that if the worst period of the current episode was actually before the past month (i.e., the depressed mood has partially remitted in the past month), the clinician should still focus on the period of the past 4 weeks to determine whether criteria are met for a current MDE. If criteria are not ultimately met, then the clinician would continue with the assessment for a past MDE, using the worst period occurring prior to the past month as a focal point.

Ratings for compound items.   Several of the MDE criteria contain multiple subcomponents (i.e., Criteria A3, A4, A5, A7, A8, and A9) some of which are polar opposites (e.g., insomnia and hypersomnia, psychomotor agitation and psychomotor retardation). A rating of "+" for such items reflects the presence of any one of the subcomponents (e.g., insomnia OR hypersomnia nearly every day during the 2-week period).

Common errors made in assessing MDEs are as follows:

- One of the most common errors made in the assessment of an MDE is the failure of the clinician to ensure that each symptom has been present nearly every day during the 2-week time frame established at the beginning of the inquiry. We therefore strongly recommend that the clinician specifically ask, "Was that true nearly every day during this period?" after each symptom, even to the point of being tediously repetitive, because there is no other way to ensure that this persistence requirement is met for each item as required by the MDE criteria set. To underscore this point, the phrase "nearly every day" is underlined as a reminder. It should not be assumed that just because the first several symptoms are present nearly every day during the 2-week time interval, each of the rest also persisted for 2 weeks—each symptom can potentially have its own independent course (e.g., sleep and appetite changes may be present nearly every day for the 2-week period in question, but fatigue and difficulty concentrating may be present for only a minority of the days). Note that Criterion A9 (recurrent thoughts of death or suicidal ideation or a suicide attempt or specific plan) is the only criterion that need *not* be present nearly every day—recurrent suicidal ideation or a single suicide attempt alone warrants a rating of "+".

- A second common error is to neglect to establish a clear 2-week time frame to reference throughout Criterion A. As noted in the beginning of Criterion A, even though the initial time frame for the current MDE inquiry is "in the past month," the actual requirement is for five (or more) of the symptoms to have been present during the same 2-week period. Neglecting to restrict the questions to a 2-week time frame will result in the patient assuming that the minimum required duration for each item is 1 month instead of only 2 weeks. Even when the clinician clearly states that the focus is only on a particular 2-week time interval, it is advisable to remind the patient of the applicable time frame at least once or twice during the course of assessing the nine Criterion A MDE items.

- A third issue that can lead to scoring errors concerns counting symptoms that occur in the context of a comorbid GMC. GMCs may manifest with the same types of symptoms that characterize a depressive episode (e.g., weight loss, insomnia, fatigue). Under what circumstances should they be attributed to the depression or the GMC? The rule in DSM-5 is to consider such symptoms as part of the MDE UNLESS they are clearly attributable to a GMC. For example, insomnia that is entirely explained by frequent nocturnal coughing spells in a person with bronchitis should not count for Criterion A4.

- A final issue is whether to consider as part of the MDE symptoms that were present before the onset of the episode (e.g., chronic insomnia). The initial part of Criterion A requires that each symptom "represent a change from previous functioning." Thus, chronic symptoms should count toward a diagnosis of an MDE only if they have become appreciably worse during the depressive episode. For example, if a patient who usually takes 30 minutes to fall asleep finds that it has been taking 2 hours to fall asleep since the episode began, it would make sense to rate Criterion A4 as present for the episode.

Criterion A1—Depressed mood.   Depressed mood may be acknowledged directly (e.g., "I've been feeling depressed" or "I can't stop crying"); by one of its many synonyms (sad, blue, tearful, empty, "down in the dumps"); or, in a new addition to DSM-5, as feelings of hopelessness. Alternatively, this criterion can be rated as present if the patient reports that others have commented that he or she has been looking depressed or down. Depressed mood in an MDE can be distinguished from "ordinary" (i.e., non-pathological) depression by virtue of its persistence and severity. To count toward this criterion, the patient's depressed mood must have been present for most of the day, nearly every day, for at least 2 weeks. Note that the criterion can be rated "+" based on observational information, even if it runs counter to the patient's report (e.g., a stoic elderly patient denies being depressed whereas the staff reports that the patient has been continuously tearful).

Criterion A2—Diminished interest or pleasure.   Although the cardinal symptom of an MDE is depressed mood, it may sometimes be diagnosed in the absence of a subjective feeling of depression. Some patients, particularly those with severe presentations, have lost the capacity to feel sadness. Others may have a cognitive style or come from a cultural setting in which feelings of sadness are downplayed. For such patients, loss of interest or pleasure counts as a "depressive equivalent" and can be substituted for depressed mood when defining the 2-week interval that applies to Criteria A3–A9. Given the dual functionality of Criterion A2 (i.e., as a depressive equivalent and as one of the nine symptoms that make up an MDE), two different wordings (linked by bracketed arrows) are provided for the question depending on which function applies. If the clinician has already established the presence of depressed mood lasting at least 2 weeks (i.e., Criterion A1 is coded "+"), then the first version of the question is asked in order to determine whether there was also diminished interest or pleasure during the previously identified period of depressed mood. If, however, no 2-week period of depressed mood has been established, then the second question is asked in order to establish whether there has been a 2-week period of diminished interest or pleasure lasting most of the day, nearly every day. Evidence of this symptom may be that the patient reports a general marked diminishing of pleasure (e.g., "nothing makes me happy anymore") or specific examples such as no longer reading books, watching TV, going to the movies, socializing with friends or family, or having sex. When rating this item, note that complete loss of interest or the ability to experience pleasure is not necessarily required for a rating of "+"; evidence that there is a significant reduction in the ability to experience pleasure will suffice.

Criterion A3—Appetite/weight change.   This item is rated "+" if there has been a significant change in appetite, either up or down, OR a significant change in weight during the 2-week target period. Given that it is relatively unusual for a significant weight change to have occurred entirely within a 2-week time frame, the SCID-5-CV asks about appetite changes first. The clinician only needs to ask about weight change if there has been no significant change in appetite. Be forewarned, however, that significant changes in weight without corresponding appetite changes suggest the possibility that a GMC may be responsible for the change in weight. Note that the first part of this item focuses on appetite and not on the amount of food consumed; thus, a rating of "+" should be made only if the patient acknowledges a significant change in his or her appetite.

Criterion A4—Sleep disturbance.   *Insomnia* may be manifested in many different ways, any one of which can count for this item. These include difficulty falling asleep, waking up a number of times in the middle of the night, and awakening much earlier than is normal for that person, with an inability to fall back asleep. *Hypersomnia* is sleeping much more than is normal for the person. In order to establish that the sleep pattern represents a change for the patient, it is important to determine the person's typical sleep pattern before the onset of the episode of depressed mood or diminished interest or pleasure. Note that it is difficult and potentially not very meaningful to establish an absolute definition of the number of hours of sleep that constitute insomnia or hypersomnia because of wide variability in individuals' need for sleep. However, as a rule of thumb, sleeping 2 hours more or less than is typical on a daily basis would constitute hypersomnia or insomnia. Note that hypersomnia should not be coded for someone who stays in bed for most of the day but is not sleeping.

Criterion A5—Psychomotor activity changes. *Psychomotor agitation and retardation* refer to changes in motor activity and rate of thinking. Although many depressed patients describe a subjective feeling of being restless or slowed down, Criterion A5 should not be counted unless the symptoms are visibly apparent to an outside observer (e.g., the patient seems to move in slow motion or is either pacing or unable to sit still). If the symptom is not currently present and observable by the clinician, there must be a convincing behavioral description of past agitation or retardation that was sufficiently severe to be observed by others. Be sure to distinguish the feelings of being slowed down in psychomotor retardation (e.g., "I feel like I'm walking through a vat of molasses") from feelings of having no motivation to do anything (coded in Criterion A2) and feelings of having no energy (coded in Criterion A6).

Criterion A6—Fatigue or loss of energy. Patients with this symptom may report feeling tired all the time, "running on low power," feeling "weak" all the time, or feeling totally drained after minimal physical activity. When a patient complains about not feeling like doing anything, the clinician should differentiate between lack of energy (Criterion A6) and loss of interest or motivation (coded in Criterion A2), which may also be present.

Criterion A7—Worthlessness/guilt. Be careful in rating this item because patients who are depressed but who do not have the full syndrome of MDE symptoms often acknowledge feeling bad about themselves or feeling guilty. The actual item requires a more severe disturbance in self-perception—either feelings of worthlessness OR excessive or inappropriate guilt. Although patients often report feeling guilty about the negative impact their problems have on others ("I feel so guilty for being such a burden"), such feelings are not considered to be examples of "excessive or inappropriate guilt" as required by the criterion. A true positive response requires evidence of exaggerated and inappropriate guilt (e.g., "I feel like I've ruined my family forever") that goes beyond self-reproach about being sick.

Criterion A8—Cognitive disturbance. Cognitive impairment in depression is sometimes severe enough to resemble dementia. With less severe, but still significant, impairment, a patient may be unable to concentrate on any activity (e.g., watching TV, reading a newspaper) due to an inability to filter out brooding thoughts. Clinicians should note that the impairment caused by this symptom may vary depending on the patient's baseline. For example, a theoretical mathematician may still be able to watch TV but no longer be able to concentrate on mathematical proofs—in such an instance, a rating of "+" would be warranted. Note that the second half of this item taps a different type of impairment (i.e., indecisiveness). A patient with this symptom may report feeling paralyzed by even simple decisions, such as which clothes to wear for the day or what to eat for lunch.

Criterion A9—Suicidal thoughts. This is the only symptom that does not need to be present nearly every day for at least 2 weeks to warrant a rating of "+". Any recurrent, active suicidal thoughts or behavior (i.e., suicidal thoughts that include a plan, intention, and means to carry out that plan) or any single suicide attempt is sufficient for a rating of "+". Having frequent thoughts of passive suicidal ideation would also warrant a "+" rating, such as: "I'd be better off dead" or "My family would be better off if I were dead." If there are current suicidal thoughts, it is imperative that the clinician determine the nature of the ideation (active or passive suicidal thoughts) and take appropriate action. Self-mutilating behavior (e.g., cutting, burning) can be an expression of anger or frustration, or aimed at controlling strong emotions. Self-harm behavior without suicidal intent is coded "—".

Criterion B—Clinical significance. DSM-5 has included this "clinical significance" criterion with most of the disorders in order to emphasize the requirement that a symptom pattern must lead to impairment or distress before being considered diagnosable as a mental disorder. In most circumstances, the fact that the symptoms have had a significant impact on the patient's life will already be known to the clinician in the course of eliciting descriptive information to support the ratings of the items making up the depressive syndrome. However, if the impact of the symptoms on the patient's functioning is unclear, additional questions are provided to help determine the impact of the symptoms on the patient's academic, occupational, and social functioning.

Criterion C—Not due to a GMC and NOT substance/medication-induced. This criterion instructs the clinician to consider and rule out a GMC or a substance/medication as an etiological factor. See Section 9, "Differentiating General Medical and Substance/Medication Etiologies From Primary Disorders," in this User's Guide for a discussion of how to rate this criterion. If the clinician decides that the diagnosis is Depressive Disorder Due to Another Medical Condition or Substance/Medication-Induced Depressive Disorder, that diagnosis should be recorded in the Diagnostic Summary Score Sheet under Depressive Disorders.

Number of episodes. After making a rating of "+" indicating that the criteria are met for a current MDE, the clinician is instructed to make a rough estimate of the total number of episodes, which is used for the later determination of whether Major Depressive Disorder is Single Episode or Recurrent. This entails asking the patient to report how many separate times he or she has had an MDE—it does not mean that the clinician must inquire about each symptom for each episode. Note that according to the DSM-5 definition of "recurrent episodes" in Major Depressive Disorder, episodes are considered to be separate if there is an interval of at least 2 consecutive months in which criteria are not met for an MDE. Thus, a symptom-free period between episodes is not required.

10.3.2.   Ratings for Past Major Depressive Episode (A15–A28)

If the symptoms do not meet criteria for a current episode, the clinician then needs to inquire in detail about past periods of depressed mood or diminished interest or pleasure. Because of the difficulty that some patients may have in recalling both the presence and temporal relationship of specific symptoms occurring years earlier, it is <u>essential</u> for the clinician to select a specific 2-week interval during the past depressive period to be the target period for the subsequent eight questions. We recommend using holidays, seasons, or other life events (e.g., birthdays, graduation) as "landmarks" to narrow down the 2-week period in which the depression was the worst. To bring that time period into sharp focus in the patient's mind, another strategy is to ask specific questions about contextual factors associated with that time of the person's life (e.g., "Where were you living at the time? Where were you working? What semester or grade were you in at school?"). The process of carefully reviewing the patient's past thus serves to transform the time period from an abstraction (i.e., "that time 10 years ago when I was depressed") to a more vivid memory so that the reporting of specific symptoms is more likely to be valid. For example, let's say a patient reports being depressed for several months during his junior year in college. The clinician may try to pinpoint a 2-week interval as follows: "I know it's hard to be this precise, but I need you to focus on a 2-week period when it was the worst. Were you depressed during the fall semester of your junior year, or in the spring?" Patient answers "spring." The clinician asks: "Was it before or after spring break?" "How close was it to finals?" and so forth. We recognize that this process can be relatively time-consuming and that some clinicians may be tempted to accept a vague time frame from the patient before embarking on the past MDE assessment. We strongly recommend investing the time and energy into establishing a firm, concrete time frame because of the likely lack of validity of the patient's answers to questions such as "During that time when you were depressed 8 years ago, how was your appetite?"

In those situations in which the patient reports more than one past episode in his or her lifetime, the clinician should establish which of the episodes was "the worst," and subsequent questions should focus on the worst 2-week period during that "worst" episode. However, there are a couple of exceptions to this rule:

1. If there has been an episode in the past year, the clinician should ask about this period first even if it was not "the worst," because it is more recent and therefore the patient is more likely to have a better memory of the symptomatic details.
2. When there are several possible episodes to choose from, it makes sense to favor episodes that occur at times during which the patient was NOT using substances/medications that are known to cause depression and NOT suffering from a potentially etiological GMC. For example, if the patient reports two past episodes, a se-

vere episode occurring during a period of heavy cocaine use and a milder episode occurring during an extended period of abstinence, the clinician should start with the latter episode (of abstinence) and consider the former episode (comorbid with the cocaine use) only if the latter episode does not meet criteria for an MDE.

REMEMBER that based on the SCID algorithm, detailed symptomatic ratings for past MDE need to be made ONLY IF the criteria are NOT met for a current MDE (i.e., either no current depressed mood or depressed mood accompanied by insufficient symptoms to meet criteria for current MDE).

Note that when the clinician asks about a past episode, the specific wording for the introductory questions in item labels A15 and A16 (i.e., "Have you _ever_ had…") should be adjusted depending on the answers to the prior introductory questions about a current period of depressed mood or diminished interest or pleasure (corresponding to Criteria A1 and A2 for current MDE, item labels A1 and A2). If either of these questions was answered "YES" (indicating that there is a current period of depressed mood or diminished interest or pleasure that ultimately did not meet full criteria for an MDE), then the clinician is instructed to substitute the phrase (italics for identification) "_Has there ever been another time_ when you were feeling depressed or down most of the day nearly every day?" for "_Have you ever had a period of time_ when…?"

When a rating of "—"or "NO" is made for any of the critical criteria when evaluating a current MDE, the clinician skips out of the evaluation of the current MDE and goes on to the evaluation of past MDE. When evaluating a past MDE and the clinician reaches a point in the evaluation when it becomes clear that the criteria are not met, if there is a history of multiple past periods of depression it is important for the clinician to consider whether one of the periods OTHER than the one selected for the evaluation of past MDE may possibly meet full criteria for an MDE before skipping out of the evaluation of past MDE and continuing with the evaluation of a current Manic Episode. Even though the clinician has presumably selected the "worst" period during the initial evaluation of past episodes, which in most cases is the one most likely to meet full criteria, there are two circumstances in which an episode other than the one selected might be more likely to meet criteria for MDE: 1) if the clinician decided to focus on an episode in the past year rather than the "worst" one in the person's life (as per SCID-5-CV instructions); or 2) if the patient's idea of which episode was the "worst" differs from the requirements of the MDE criteria (i.e., the patient selected an episode that was the most distressing but had relatively few symptoms or a minimal impact on functioning).

The questions covering the nine items making up Criterion A for past MDE are identical in content to their counterparts in current MDE except that they are worded in the past tense.

Rating Current Major Depressive Episode, In Partial Remission, as a past episode. Sometimes a patient is interviewed with the SCID-5-CV at a point in time during which an MDE is partially remitted. For example, 2 months ago the patient may have been depressed with persistent loss of interest, insomnia, poor appetite, low energy, and thoughts of suicide. At the time of the SCID-5-CV interview, his depressed mood and loss of interest persist, but he is now sleeping better, his appetite is back, and he no longer thinks of suicide. Thus, when the clinician is evaluating current MDE in the SCID-5-CV, the patient's symptoms would not meet criteria for current MDE (past month). However, when the clinician is evaluating past MDE, the patient's symptoms would meet criteria for past MDE (with an onset of 2 months ago). On the Diagnostic Summary Score Sheet, such a patient's condition would be diagnosed as Major Depressive Disorder, In Partial Remission.

10.3.3   Ratings for Current Manic Episode (A29–A40)

Remember that for the purposes of the SCID, "current" refers to the entire past month so that the patient does not need to appear manic during the interview to be diagnosed as having a current Manic Episode.

Criterion A.   *Criterion A (Part I)—Abnormally elevated or irritable mood + increased activity or energy.*   Criterion A has been split into two separate parts in the SCID-5-CV to allow the diagnoses of both Manic Episode and Hypomanic Episode to be ruled out if the first part of the criterion is not present. The first part (item label A29) establishes that there has been a distinct period of abnormally elevated, expansive, or irritable mood accompanied by increased activity or energy that has lasted for at least several days, a required feature of both a Manic Episode and a Hypomanic Episode. (The bracketed phrase "lasting at least several days," which is not actually part of the DSM-5 criterion, has been added to provide a minimum duration of symptoms in order to justify skipping out of the assessment of a <u>current</u> Manic and Hypomanic Episode if this item is rated "—".) This criterion reflects the DSM-5 requirement that there be an abnormally and persistently elevated, expansive, or irritable mood <u>combined with</u> persistently increased activity or energy.

To ensure that clinicians do not neglect to inquire about irritable mood, the inquiry about irritability has been formulated into a separate question (i.e., "Have you had a period of time when you were feeling irritable, angry, or short-tempered for most of the day, for at least several days?"). Patients often describe periods of irritability that are either an associated feature of an MDE or chronic irritability that is a symptom of a personality disturbance. Irritability that is indicative of a true Manic Episode is abnormally intense for that person (e.g., a maniacal ranting at a customer service representative, in contrast to merely being "snippy" with his or her spouse) and by definition must be accompanied by increased activity or energy, features not typically seen in an irritable depression or a personality disorder. However, if there is any question whether the irritability might be part of a Manic or Hypomanic Episode, the clinician should continue to ask all the manic (or hypomanic) symptom questions in order to make a judgment as to whether the irritability is a symptom of a Manic or Hypomanic Episode or is better accounted for by another condition like depression.

Criterion A (Part II)—1-week duration.   The criteria sets for Manic and Hypomanic Episode are symptomatically identical but differ in terms of minimum duration (Manic Episode has a minimum duration of 1 week whereas Hypomanic Episode has a minimum duration of only 4 days) and severity (Manic Episodes cause significant impairment in functioning whereas Hypomanic Episodes by definition must NOT cause significant impairment). The second part of Criterion A (item label A30) serves to differentiate between the two episodes based on duration (i.e., if the duration of the elevated/irritable mood is less than 1 week, then the clinician is instructed to skip to item label A41 to check for a current Hypomanic Episode). Note that an episode duration of less than 1 week would qualify for a Manic Episode if the episode is sufficiently severe to require hospitalization.

The separate questions for the evaluation of elevated mood and irritable mood can potentially result in a diagnostic algorithm error if the following sequence of questions occurs:

- Clinician asks the patient about whether there has been a distinct period of abnormally elevated or euphoric mood plus increased activity or energy.
- Patient answers "YES," justifying a rating of "+" on the first part of Criterion A.
- Clinician then asks the patient about duration.
- Patient indicates that the period of elevated mood has lasted for only 5 days (without hospitalization) so the clinician skips to the evaluation of current Hypomanic Episode (ruling out a diagnosis of a current Manic Episode).

In this sequence, the presence of a distinct period of irritable mood is not known to the clinician (the question about irritability was not asked, given the patient's initial positive response to the question about elevated mood). It is possible that the patient might have had a period of abnormally irritable mood plus increased activity or energy that lasted 1 week or more, justifying the continued evaluation of the criteria for a Manic Episode. Thus, a *NOTE* has been included in the SCID-5-CV under Part II of Criterion A, instructing the clinician to be sure to check for irritable mood lasting at least 1 week before skipping out of the evaluation of current Manic Episode (i.e., "If elevated mood lasts less than 1 week, check whether there has been a period of irritable mood lasting at least 1 week before skipping to **A41**").

It is essential to identify a 1-week time frame within the past month in order to ensure that the manic symptoms co-occur during the same 1-week period (similar to the evaluation of a current MDE, which requires symptoms to co-occur within an identified 2-week period). The clinician therefore starts the evaluation by asking the patient when, during the past month, he or she was the most manic. If the severity was relatively the same throughout the past month, then the most recent week should be used as the time frame.

Criterion B.   It is important to remember that in order to count a Criterion B symptom toward the diagnosis of a Manic Episode, the symptom must be present during the period of elevated or irritable mood and must be persistent and clinically significant.

Criterion B1—Inflated self-esteem or grandiosity.   The grandiosity or inflated self-esteem is clearly not justified; merely being more self-confident than usual would not suffice for a rating of "+".

Criterion B2—Decreased need for sleep.   The patient should report feeling rested after only a few hours of sleep in order to justify a rating of "+" for this Criterion B item. The prototypical patient feels that he or she does not need to sleep at all and describes feeling driven or "wired" and cannot calm down enough to sleep. It is important to distinguish Criterion B2 from insomnia—while both are characterized by sleeping fewer hours than usual, with insomnia that individual wants to be able to sleep, but is unable to sleep and feels tired the next day.

Criterion B3—More talkative or pressure to keep talking.   The increase in talkativeness is manifest in both the rate and amount of speech. The speech often has a driven quality, as if there is so much to say and not nearly enough time to say it. If present during the interview, it may be very difficult for the clinician to interrupt the patient's monologue.

Criterion B4—Flight of ideas or racing thoughts.   This criterion can be rated "+" based either on the patient's subjective report that his or her thoughts are racing OR on the clinical judgment that flight of ideas has been present (based either on observation of the patient's pattern of thinking or by history). Flight of ideas involves thoughts that are loosely connected, with the patient jumping from one topic to another very quickly, with only the slightest thread of thematic connection between topics. In some cases, the connection may be based on sound rather than meaning (clang association).

Criterion B5—Distractibility.   Distractibility refers to an inability to filter out extraneous stimuli (i.e., stimuli external to the person) while attempting to focus on a particular task. For example, the patient may have trouble focusing on the clinician's questions because of being distracted by a police siren on the street, and may need to jump up from the interview and investigate what is going on outside. Being distracted by one's own racing thoughts would not by itself justify a rating of "+".

Criterion B6—Increased goal-directed activity or psychomotor agitation.   As a consequence of elevated mood, increased energy, or increased self-esteem, the patient may become involved in more goal-directed activities than usual either socially, at work or school, or sexually. Typical "manic" activities involve calling friends at all hours of the night, beginning new creative projects, or being more sexually active. Alternatively, the increase in activity may be more diffuse and be manifest as psychomotor agitation (i.e., purposeless non-goal-directed activity, such as pacing or being unable to sit still).

Criterion B7—Excessive involvement in risky activities.   In the pursuit of pleasure, excitement, or thrills, or simply the bad judgment characteristic of mania, the person may engage in activities that are uncharacteristic of him or her, without regard to possible negative consequences. Typical examples include spending large sums of money on luxury items or services, gifts for others, or expensive vacations; engaging in sexual indiscretions; reckless driving; or foolish or risky business investments.

Must have three (or more) symptoms, four if mood is only irritable. The number of items required to meet Criterion B depends on whether Criterion A was coded "+" on the basis of euphoric mood or on irritable mood only. If euphoric mood has been present, then only three Criterion B items need to have been present. Irritable mania requires a minimum of four Criterion B items to help differentiate it from irritable MDEs.

Criterion C—Causing marked impairment, requiring hospitalization, or psychotic symptoms. A comparison of the criteria for Manic and Hypomanic Episodes reveals that these two entities share the same symptoms, but differ in minimum duration and the degree of severity. As indicated in this criterion, the symptoms in a Manic Episode must be sufficiently severe so as to cause marked impairment in functioning, require hospitalization, or include psychotic features. Otherwise, a diagnosis of Hypomanic Episode should be considered (and in most cases, would be warranted if the clinician has reached this point in the criteria list). For this reason, if a rating of "—" is made for Criterion C (item label A39), the clinician is instructed to skip to the criteria for current Hypomanic Episode, picking up with Criterion C, item label A50 (because meeting Criteria A and B for Manic Episode necessarily means that the corresponding Criteria A and B in Hypomanic Episode are also met).

Criterion D—Not due to a GMC or substance/medication-induced. This criterion instructs the clinician to consider and rule out a GMC or a substance/medication as an etiological factor. See Section 9, "Differentiating General Medical and Substance/Medication Etiologies From Primary Disorders," in this User's Guide for a discussion of how to rate this criterion. If the clinician decides that the diagnosis is Bipolar and Related Disorder Due to Another Medical Condition or Substance/Medication-Induced Bipolar and Related Disorder, that diagnosis should be recorded in the Diagnostic Summary Score Sheet.

Note that Manic Episodes that are triggered by somatic antidepressant treatment (including bright light therapy and electroconvulsive therapy) and that persist beyond the physiological effects of that treatment, which were considered to be substance/medication-induced under the rules of DSM-IV, are instead considered to be bona fide Manic Episodes in DSM-5. Thus, this criterion should be rated "YES" for such episodes.

10.3.4   Ratings for Current Hypomanic Episode (A41–A53)

Criterion A—Mood disturbance + increased activity or energy lasting 4 days. The only way to reach this point in the SCID-5-CV is to have skipped out of the assessment of Manic Episode as part of the evaluation of Part II of Criterion A (i.e., there was a "+" rating on the first part of Criterion A for Manic Episode, indicating a period of euphoric, elevated, or irritable mood plus increased activity or energy lasting for several days; then there was a "—" rating on the second part of Criterion A, indicating that the duration fell short of the 1-week minimum needed for a Manic Episode). In most cases, to evaluate this criterion the clinician need only to determine whether the mood disturbance + increased activity or energy lasted for at least 4 consecutive days.

Because there could have been several hypomanic periods lasting at least 4 days in the past month, the clinician is instructed to determine which one was the "most severe" and then to focus on that period for the remaining questions in this section.

Criterion B—Syndrome of hypomanic symptoms. By definition, a Hypomanic Episode is severe enough to be distinguishable from "normal" good mood (see Criteria C and D) but not so severe that it causes marked functional impairment (see Criterion E). As can be seen with this criterion, the description of the specific hypomanic symptoms is identical in wording to that in the definition of a Manic Episode and is differentiated solely based on severity. Please refer to the annotations for the Criterion B items in Section 10.3.3, "Ratings for Current Manic Episode," of this User's Guide for more information.

Criterion C—Unequivocal change in functioning. To rate this criterion "+", the clinician must ensure that mood change and other symptoms result in a clear-cut change in functioning (e.g., increased productivity at work) that is not typical of the person's functioning when not in an episode.

Criterion D—Observable by others. To further ensure that the mood change is significant, this criterion requires that the change in functioning be observable by others—a subjective sense of elevated mood that is not corroborated by others does not count. In lieu of information from informants, examples of situations in which others commented about the patient's change in behavior are acceptable.

Criterion E—Absence of marked impairment. This criterion is the opposite of Criterion C in Manic Episode and requires that the hypomanic symptoms not be severe enough to cause marked functional impairment or necessitate hospitalization and that there are no psychotic symptoms. If the hypomanic symptoms are sufficiently severe to cause marked impairment, lead to hospitalization, or involve psychotic symptoms, then Criterion E should be rated "—", ruling out a diagnosis of a current Hypomanic Episode. In such cases, the clinician is instructed to return to the assessment of current Manic Episode, resuming with item label A31 (Criterion B), and to transcribe the current Hypomanic Episode Criterion B symptom ratings (item labels A42–A48) to the current Manic Episode Criterion B symptom ratings (item labels A31–A37) and then code "+" for the current Manic Episode Criterion C (item label A39) to indicate that the symptoms were sufficiently severe to cause marked impairment or necessitate hospitalization or that there were psychotic symptoms.

Criterion F—Not due to a GMC or substance/medication-induced. This criterion instructs the clinician to consider and rule out a GMC or a substance/medication as an etiological factor. See Section 9, "Differentiating General Medical and Substance/Medication Etiologies From Primary Disorders," in this User's Guide for a discussion of how to rate this criterion. If the clinician decides that the diagnosis is Bipolar and Related Disorder Due to Another Medical Condition or Substance/Medication-Induced Bipolar and Related Disorder, that diagnosis should be recorded in the Diagnostic Summary Score Sheet.

Note that Hypomanic Episodes that are triggered by somatic antidepressant treatment (including bright light therapy and electroconvulsive therapy) and that persist beyond the physiological effects of that treatment are NOT considered to be substance/medication-induced as they were under the rules of DSM-IV but are instead considered to be bona fide Hypomanic Episodes under the rules of DSM-5. Thus, this criterion should be rated "YES" for such episodes.

10.3.5 Ratings for Past Manic and Hypomanic Episodes (A54–A77)

If the criteria are met for a current Manic Episode, there is no need to assess whether there are any past Manic Episodes because only one Manic Episode in the patient's lifetime is needed to establish a diagnosis of Bipolar I Disorder. However, if criteria are not met for a current Manic Episode but are met for a current Hypomanic Episode, it is still necessary to see if the criteria for a past Manic Episode have been met in order to establish the presence of Bipolar I Disorder instead of Bipolar II Disorder.

As was the case with the assessment of past MDEs, when assessing past Manic and/or Hypomanic Episodes, it is essential for the clinician to pick a specific time interval (1 week for Manic Episode, 4 days for Hypomanic Episode) to be the target period for the subsequent seven questions. We recommend using holidays, seasons, or other life events (e.g., birthdays, graduation) as "landmarks" to narrow down the time period in which the manic/hypomanic symptoms were the most severe. Another strategy is to ask specific questions about contextual factors associated with that time of the patient's life in order to bring that period of time into sharp focus in his or her mind (e.g., "Where were you living at the time? Where were you working? What semester or grade were you in at school?"). The process of carefully reviewing the patient's past thus serves to transform the time period from an abstraction (i.e., "that time 10 years ago when I was wired and on top of the world") to a more vivid memory so that the reporting of specific symptoms is more likely to be valid.

In those situations in which the patient reports more than one past manic or hypomanic period, the clinician should establish which of the periods was the most intense and subsequent questions should focus on the most severe 1-week period (for Manic Episode) or 4-day period for Hypomanic Episode. However, there are a couple of exceptions to this rule:

1. If there has been a Manic or Hypomanic Episode in the past year, the clinician should ask about this period even if it was not the most intense period in the patient's lifetime because it is more recent; and therefore, the patient is more likely to have a better memory of the symptomatic details.
2. When there are several possible episodes to choose from, it makes sense to favor episodes that have occurred at times during which the patient was NOT using sub-

stances or medications that are known to cause mania or hypomania and was NOT suffering from a potentially etiological GMC. For example, if the patient reports two past episodes, a severe episode occurring during a period of heavy cocaine use and a milder episode occurring during an extended period of abstinence, the clinician should start with the latter episode (of abstinence) and consider the former episode (comorbid with the cocaine use) only if the latter episode does not meet criteria for a Manic or Hypomanic Episode.

Note that when the clinician asks about a past episode, the specific wording for the introductory questions in item label A54 (i.e. "Have you _ever_ had…") should be adjusted depending on the answers to the prior introductory questions about a current period of elevated mood or irritable mood (corresponding to the first part of Criterion A for current Manic or Hypomanic Episode—item label A29). If either of the questions was answered "YES" (indicating that there is a current period of elevated mood or irritable mood that ultimately did not meet full criteria for a Manic or Hypomanic Episode), then the clinician is instructed to substitute the phrase (italics for identification) "_Has there ever been another time when you were feeling so good, 'high,' excited, or 'on top of the world' that other people thought you were not your normal self?_" instead of "_Have you ever had a period of time when…?_"

In evaluating a current Manic or Hypomanic Episode, when a rating of "—" is made for any of the critical criteria, the clinician skips out of the evaluation of the current episode and on to the evaluation of past episodes. When evaluating a past Manic or Hypomanic Episode and the clinician reaches a point in the evaluation when it becomes clear that the criteria are not met, if there is a history of multiple past periods of mania or hypomania it is important for the clinician to consider whether one of the periods OTHER than the one selected may possibly meet full criteria for a Manic or Hypomanic Episode before skipping out of this section altogether and continuing with the evaluation of Persistent Depressive Disorder. Even though the clinician had presumably selected the most intense manic or hypomanic period, because in most cases that is the one most likely to meet full criteria, there are two circumstances in which an episode other than the one originally selected might be more likely to meet full criteria for a Manic or Hypomanic Episode: 1) if the clinician decided to initially focus on an episode that occurred in the past year rather than on the most severe one in the person's life (as per SCID instructions); or 2) the patient's sense of which episode was the most intense differs from the symptomatic requirements of the Manic or Hypomanic Episode criteria (i.e., the patient selected an episode that was the most memorable but had relatively few symptoms or a minimal impact on functioning). Therefore, if there is another past manic or hypomanic period that might possibly have met full criteria for a Manic or Hypomanic Episode, the clinician should go back and re-ask the manic or hypomanic questions for that period of time.

The questions covering the seven items making up Criterion B for past Manic or Hypomanic Episode are identical in content to their counterparts in current Manic or Hypomanic Episode except that they are worded in the past tense.

10.3.6   Ratings for Current Persistent Depressive Disorder (A78–A90)

Because the diagnosis of Persistent Depressive Disorder is not made if there has ever been a Manic or Hypomanic Episode, there is an instruction to skip to the assessment of psychotic symptoms (item label B1) if criteria have ever been met for a Manic or Hypomanic Episode. Although in Persistent Depressive Disorder, Criterion A (depressed mood, more days than not for 2 years), Criterion B (at least two out of six associated depressive symptoms like appetite changes and low self-esteem), and Criterion C (never without symptoms for more than 2 months at a time) are the same as their counterparts in DSM-IV Dysthymic Disorder, this DSM-5 category is not equivalent to DSM-IV Dysthymic Disorder because there is no longer any exclusion for concurrent MDEs. According to DSM-5, Persistent Depressive Disorder is diagnosed for any chronic depressive picture lasting at least 2 years—thus, any combination of mild depressive symptoms and MDEs is covered by this diagnostic entry. Three such configurations are specifically included: 1) a "pure" dysthymic presentation in which there is depressed mood, for more days than not, that is never severe enough to meet criteria for a full MDE; 2) an MDE that has lasted continuously for 2 years (which would have been specified as "chronic" in DSM-IV); and 3) a mixture of baseline dysthymic symptoms and superimposed MDEs (sometimes referred to as "double depression"). In DSM-5, Criterion D of Persistent Depressive Disorder indicates that a continuous MDE lasting at least 2 years can qualify for this diagnosis ("Criteria for a major depressive disorder may be continuously present for 2 years"; p. 168). However, because this statement does not actually function as a true diagnostic criterion (it is neither an essential feature for the diagnosis of Persistent Depressive Disorder nor an exclusion criterion) and thus cannot be meaningfully rated in the SCID-5-CV, it has been omitted. Note that Criterion F indicates that Persistent Depressive Disorder is not diagnosed if the symptoms are better explained by a psychotic disorder. Information obtained in the Overview may be sufficient for rating Criterion F; however, because psychotic disorders are not diagnosed until later in the SCID-5-CV (i.e., in Module C), it may be necessary to rate Criterion F provisionally and return to this point (item label A88) once a psychotic disorder has been more definitively ruled in or ruled out.

10.4   Module B.   Psychotic and Associated Symptoms

Module B is for assessing the lifetime occurrence of psychotic symptoms (e.g., delusions, hallucinations) and from that information determining which psychotic disorder diagnosis best applies. (Note that the term "psychotic disorders" in the SCID-5-CV includes the Schizophrenia Spectrum and Other Psychotic Disorders [excluding Schizotypal Personality Disorder] and Bipolar and Major Depressive Disorders With Psychotic Features.) Ratings for the specific criteria are contained in Module C (i.e., ratings for Schizophrenia, Schizophreniform Disorder, Schizoaffective Disorder, Delusional Disorder, Brief Psychotic Disorder, Psychotic Disorder Due to Another Medical Condition, Substance/Medication-Induced Psychotic Disorder, and Other Specified Psychotic Disorder) and Module D (i.e., ratings for Bipolar I Disorder With Psychotic

Features, Bipolar II Disorder With Psychotic Features, and Major Depressive Disorder With Psychotic Features).

Module B serves as both a checklist for recording psychotic symptoms that have emerged during the course of the SCID-5-CV interview, as well as a lifetime screener for the various types of psychotic symptoms that define the psychotic disorders in DSM-5. For most patients with a psychotic disorder, the presence of a current psychotic symptom has usually been established before Module B (usually in the Overview). If a patient is too psychotic or disorganized to sit through the SCID-5-CV interview, the evidence for psychotic symptoms will need to come from medical records or informants. In these instances, Module B may serve more as a checklist for recording those psychotic symptoms than as an interview guide. In fact, this is the one part of the SCID-5-CV where the rule requiring the clinician to paraphrase a question into a confirmatory statement if the answer is already known does not necessarily apply, because summarizing the patient's psychotic phenomenon in the form of the paraphrased screening question may be excessively off-putting to the patient and might negatively impact rapport. For example, if during the Overview the clinician has already established that the patient believes that he is God, there is no need to confirm the presence of a grandiose delusion by saying to the patient, "You've told me that you are especially important in some way or that you have special powers or knowledge."

As noted in the box immediately at the start of Module B (at the top of page 31, preceding item label B1), before rating a psychotic symptom "+", it is important for the clinician to determine whether there is a possible or definite etiological substance (including medications) or GMC. Consequently, the clinician should follow up any acknowledged psychotic symptom with some of the suggested questions to make this determination. The clinician first needs to establish whether the patient was using substances, taking medication, or ill with a GMC at the time of the onset of the psychotic symptoms with the following questions: "Just before (PSYCHOTIC SXS) began, were you using drugs?...On any medications?...Did you drink much more than usual or stop drinking after you had been drinking a lot for a while?...Were you physically ill?" If the answer to any of these questions is "YES," the clinician should follow up by determining the temporal relationship between the psychotic symptoms and the substance/medications/GMC with the following question: "Has there been a time when you had (PSYCHOTIC SXS) and were not (using [DRUG]/taking [MEDICATION]/ changing your drinking habits/physically ill)?"

When used as a screener, each of the Module B questions should be asked verbatim except if the answer to that specific question is already known. For each question answered "YES," the first step is to determine whether or not the response represents the particular psychotic symptom (e.g., a specific type of delusional belief). Thus, it is essential to ask multiple follow-up questions that are designed to elicit, in an open-ended way, the details of the patient's belief or experience in order to determine evidence of a psychotic symptom. In order to reduce the risk of false negatives, many of these questions are written quite broadly, with the understanding that they are likely to elicit positive responses in those who are not psychotic. For example, the question for persecutory delusions asks the patient "What about anyone going out of their way to give you a hard time, or trying to hurt you?" Many individuals who have had an acquaintance, coworker, or supervisor who is mean or vindictive will answer "YES" to this question. The clinician therefore needs to ask additional detailed questions to elicit sufficient information to allow for a differentiation between a realistic scenario that is not likely evidence of a delusion and a scenario that strains credulity (e.g., the belief that one's entire coterie of coworkers has been meeting off-hours at a secret location to plan ways to harass the individual) and thus suggests the presence of a persecutory delusion. As a general rule, when trying to determine whether or not a particular incident is evidence of psychosis, the clinician should give the patient the benefit of the doubt; a "+" should be coded only when the clinician is satisfied that the scenario is evidence of psychosis.

For each item coded "+", the clinician should record a description of the symptom (e.g., "is convinced that CIA has implanted a listening device into his ear"), its frequency (e.g., "daily, several times a day"), its impact on the patient's life ("e.g., "generally able to ignore this belief"), and when it occurred ("2 years ago").

It is essential to ask all patients, especially those who have already reported psychotic symptoms, all of the psychosis screening questions in Module B because they are useful both to screen generally for psychotic symptoms and to determine the full range, lifetime duration, and course of psychotic symptoms in individuals with a psychotic disorder. The same principle applies to the ratings for those psychotic symptoms that have multiple questions corresponding to the rating. So, for example, even though the delusion of reference item (item label B1) includes five questions covering various types of referential experiences, it is important to ask about each one so that the full duration and impact on the patient's life of delusions of reference can be determined.

10.4.1   Ratings of Delusions (B1–B13)

A *delusion* is a fixed false personal belief based on incorrect inference about external reality that is firmly sustained despite what almost everyone else believes and despite what constitutes incontrovertible and obvious proof or evidence to the contrary. The belief is not one ordinarily accepted by other members of the person's culture or subculture (e.g., the belief in some cultures that an individual can communicate with a dead person). When the clinician is unfamiliar with the beliefs characteristic of the patient's cultural or religious background, consultation with someone who is familiar with the patient's culture may be required to avoid the overdiagnosis of delusions.

A delusion involves impairment in the ability to make accurate logical inferences. Individuals experiencing delusional thinking draw incorrect conclusions from observations of their environment (e.g., believing that occasional phone hang-ups prove that they are the subject of an FBI surveillance operation). In rating each type of delusion, the clinician must differentiate a delusion (which would warrant a rating of "+") from a strongly held "overvalued" idea (which would warrant a rating of "—"). In deciding whether a belief is false and fixed enough to be considered a delusion, the clinician must first determine that a serious error in inference and reality testing has occurred and then determine the strength of the conviction. It may be helpful to ask the patient to talk at length about his or her conviction because it is often only in the specific details that the errors of inference become apparent. In evaluating the strength of the delusional conviction, the clinician should present alternative explanations (e.g., is it possible that the phone hang-ups are due to someone dialing a wrong number?). A patient with delusions may acknowledge the possibility of these explanations but will still hold firm to his or her own belief.

Some patients with a long-standing history of psychotic disorder have developed insight into the "psychotic" nature of their beliefs (i.e., they understand that their beliefs are a product of mental illness rather than a true reflection of reality). Such beliefs would still be considered delusions as long as, at some earlier point, they were experienced by the patient as real. For example, a patient may report that his chronic conviction that people at work are plotting against him is a result of his long-standing Schizophrenia. This would be coded as a delusion if the patient either reports that initially he was convinced the plot was real or if there is such evidence from prior records (e.g., an admission note documenting that he acted on his belief).

Types of delusions.   The first set of symptom ratings in Module B (Psychotic and Associated Symptoms) inquires about the lifetime occurrence of the various types of delusions, based on theme and content. Note that more than one rating may apply for a particular delusion if the content of the delusion covers several themes. For example, a patient who believes that the FBI is after him because he can control other people's minds would receive a rating of "+" for both persecutory and grandiose types of delusions.

Delusion of reference.   There is a relatively high false-positive response rate to the initial question for this type of delusion ("Has it ever seemed like people were talking about you or taking special notice of you?") because it asks about such a common experience. The clinician should therefore ask for specific examples that establish the psychotic nature of the belief. Most people have at some time felt that other people were talking about them, particularly if they have some obvious physical abnormality or act in a way that makes them stand out. It is therefore important to differentiate realistic perceptions, social anxiety, or transient suspiciousness from a fixed false belief. A homeless man who dresses in rags and has no place to take a shower may realistically believe that people are moving away from him on the subway, but if he believes that today's headlines are a cryptic reference to his personal life, the clinician should rate this item a "+". Because delusions of reference can be manifested in a variety of situations, a number of additional questions are provided covering a range of stimuli that are often misinterpreted as having personal significance, such as believing that something on the radio, on a TV program, or in a movie; the words to a popular song; the clothes that people are wearing; or what is written on signs or billboards was intended to send the person a special message.

Persecutory delusion.   As noted earlier, the clinician should take care to differentiate an exaggerated, but possibly valid, perception of persecution (e.g., by a boss, a teacher, an ex-spouse, a drug dealer) from a real persecutory delusion. The two follow-up questions ("Have you ever had the feeling that you were being followed, spied on, manipulated, or plotted against?" and "Did you ever have the feeling that you were being poisoned or that your food had been tampered with?") can be helpful in identifying the more obvious cases.

Grandiose delusion.   It is sometimes hard to tell where a patient's inflated perception of one's talents ends and a grandiose delusion begins. A taxi driver who believes he will write a best-selling novel may be mistaken but is not necessarily delusional. If, however, he tells the clinician that Steven Spielberg has been calling him and begging for the movie rights to his novel, he has probably stepped over the line into delusion. Questioning him about his evidence for the belief is a good way to clarify the issue.

Somatic delusion.   In assessing this symptom, it is necessary to take into account the patient's understanding of anatomy and physiology. An uneducated person may have a primitive explanation of symptoms, for example, believing that stomach pains are caused by a grasshopper hopping around inside him. A willingness to entertain an alternative explanation indicates that the belief is not a delusion. Another example of a potential false positive would be a patient with physical symptoms who is convinced that she is dying of an undiagnosed fatal illness and doubts an internist's reassurance that there is nothing medically wrong with her. If the patient is able to entertain the possibility that her concerns are exaggerated, then the diagnosis would be Somatic Symptom Disorder or Illness Anxiety Disorder. A patient who repeatedly dismisses such reassurances out of hand is more likely to have a somatic delusion. Note that a patient's delusional belief that a part of his or her body is ugly or defective is no longer recorded as a somatic delusion but instead is considered to be evidence for Body Dysmorphic Disorder, With Absent Insight.

Delusion of guilt.   This type of delusion involves a patient's belief that a minor error in the past will lead to disaster, that he or she has committed a horrible crime and should be punished severely, or that he or she is responsible for a disaster (e.g., an earthquake or fire) for which there can be no possible connection. Consequently, three questions have been included covering having committed a crime, having done something that would result in harm to others, and being responsible for a disaster. Because it is certainly possible for a patient to have been responsible for hurting others, the clinician must obtain sufficient details to establish the credibility of the patient's belief that he or she was responsible.

Jealous delusion.   The essential feature of this delusion is that the patient's sexual partner is unfaithful. For example, when asked about jealous delusions, a patient may respond that his wife is having an affair with the next-door neighbor. The clinician's task is to determine the plausibility of these claims (e.g., what did the patient see or hear to give him that impression, has anyone else observed the partner being unfaithful). Again, distinguishing a jealous delusion from concerns justified by the partner's behavior can be challenging. Usually the judgment that a belief is evidence of psychosis depends on details of the person's belief stretching the bounds of believability (e.g., a patient's belief that her husband is having sex with a mistress during the 3 minutes in which he is outside taking out the trash).

Religious delusion.   This item should be coded "+" if the content of the delusion involves religious or spiritual content. Distinguishing a religious delusion from a religious belief can be particularly challenging. One of the elements of the DSM-5 glossary definition of delusion (included above item label B1) is that the belief be <u>false</u>; this standard cannot be applied to religious beliefs because they cannot be proven to be either true or false. Instead, the method suggested in DSM-5 for deciding whether a religious belief is likely to be delusional is to determine whether or not the belief is something that is ordinarily accepted by other members of that person's religious community as a part of that religion's canon of beliefs.

Given the contextual importance of the patient's spiritual worldview, the first question is intended to determine whether the patient considers himself or herself to be a religious or spiritual person. If so, the follow-up question asks whether the patient has ever had any religious or spiritual experiences that others in his or her religious circle have not experienced. If so, then the patient is asked to describe those experiences, as well as the reactions of other members of his or her religious community to those beliefs. If the patient has not shared these beliefs with others, then it will be up to the clinician to make the determination about whether these beliefs significantly deviate from the norm dictated by the patient's religious circle. If the clinician is not familiar enough with the patient's religion to be able to make such a judgment, it may be necessary for the clinician to speak with others who are members of the patient's religion or to consult with other outside sources in order to determine whether the patient's belief falls within the norm. If the patient denies having any beliefs that are not shared by others in his or her community, then the clinician asks whether the patient has ever directly communicated with "God, the devil, or some other spiritual being or higher power." Because such communication is an experience common to a number of religions, it is essential for the clinician to determine whether such direct communication deviates from the religious norm. For those patients who report such beliefs but who have never been religious or spiritual before having those beliefs, the details of how these beliefs arose may be more indicative of a delusional process.

Erotomanic delusion.   With this type of delusion, the patient is convinced that another person, usually of higher status, is in love with him or her. For example, when asked about erotomanic delusions, a patient may respond that she "knows" that a specific celebrity is secretly in love with her but that when the patient tried to make contact, the celebrity denied even knowing her. In some cases, the patient will simply assert that he has been romantically involved with someone famous or powerful. Of course, because this could feasibly be true, it is essential to elicit as many details as possible about the relationship in order to assess whether it is fantasy or reality.

Delusion of being controlled.   With this type of delusion the patient experiences his or her feelings, impulses, thoughts, or actions as being under the direct control of some external force rather than under his or her own control. Because individuals with such delusions usually report this as something they are experiencing rather than as a belief, the SCID question is framed in terms of ever having had such a feeling. However, this item should be coded "+" (i.e., it represents a delusion) only if the patient is convinced that this experience is real. It is important to avoid confusing the colloquial experience of being in a controlling relationship as evidence of this delusion. For example, when asked about delusions of control, a patient may respond that her mother is always trying to control her. It is up to the clinician to determine whether she is talking about her actions or thoughts being controlled in some mysterious way (a true delusion of control) or whether she is simply describing a chronic struggle with her mother about what she is and is not allowed to do (probably not a delusion of any kind).

Thought insertion and thought withdrawal.   As with delusions of control, some patients with Schizophrenia may have the experience of their thoughts being controlled by some sort of outside influence. Specifically, this might entail feeling that thoughts have been inserted into their mind or that thoughts have been removed from their brain. As with delusions of being controlled, a rating of "+" should be given (i.e., they represent delusions) only if the person is convinced that these experiences are real.

Thought broadcasting.   This delusion involves the patient's feeling that his or her thoughts are being broadcast out loud so that they can be perceived by others. This item is coded "+" <u>only</u> if the patient is convinced that these experiences are real. It may be helpful to ask the patient for an explanation of how this may be happening, as a delusional interpretation of the experience ("a thought transmitter has been surgically implanted in my head") usually justifies a rating of "+". However, a recounting of the mechanism is not necessarily required for a rating of "+", as long as the patient reports these experiences as being real. If the patient experiences the broadcast thoughts as a hallucination (i.e., the patient can hear his or her thoughts as well), the item for auditory hallucinations (item label B14) should be also rated "+". Note that thought broadcasting is not the same as the more commonly reported experience that others can read one's mind, which would be coded under the next item, "Other delusions."

Other delusions.   This item is for rating delusions whose content is not covered by any of the above items, such as the patient's belief that others can read his or her mind; a nihilistic delusion (i.e., that everything, including the self, does not exist); or the related delusion that he or she has already died.

10.4.2   Ratings of Hallucinations (B14–B19)

A *hallucination* is the experience of sensory perception without stimulation of the relevant sensory organ. A hallucination should be distinguished from an illusion, which is the misperception of an actual stimulus (e.g., misinterpreting a shadow as the figure of a man).

Types of hallucinations. *Auditory hallucinations.* Auditory hallucinations should be differentiated from delusions of reference, in which the patient hears real voices (e.g., on the street, on the ward) and interprets them self-referentially (e.g., "they are talking about me"). Evidence that they are, in fact, hallucinations might be that they occur when the patient is alone. This item should be coded "+" only if the hallucinations are judged to be clinically significant (i.e., recurrent or persistent). Hearing one's name being called and finding no one there is an example of a hallucination that is not clinically significant.

Visual, tactile, somatic, gustatory, and olfactory hallucinations. Visual hallucinations must be distinguished from illusions, which are misperceptions of real stimuli (e.g., mistaking a pile of clothes in a dimly lit room for an animal). Visual phenomena during the transition to and from wakefulness and sleep (hypnagogic and hypnopompic hallucinations) should be coded "—". Tactile hallucinations involve sensations that are perceived through the surface of the skin, like being stroked or the feeling of crawling insects. Somatic hallucinations involve sensations perceived to be inside the body, like a feeling of electricity. Gustatory hallucinations, which involve the sense of taste, and olfactory hallucinations, which involve the sense of smell, can be challenging to differentiate from the patient having a particularly acute sense of taste or smell, given that the questions are framed in terms of tasting or smelling things that no one else can taste or smell. The details of the experience (e.g., persistence in multiple situations) and the nature of the smell or taste (e.g., rotting flesh, gasoline) might be especially suggestive of an hallucinatory experience.

10.4.3 Ratings for Disorganized Speech and Behavior and Catatonia (B20–B22)

Disorganized speech. Although current disorganized speech is assessed during the course of the SCID interview, past instances must be determined by history and almost always require an informant. If the patient's current speech is disorganized enough to warrant a rating of "+", it may be difficult or impossible to administer the SCID-5-CV. The assessment of this criterion requires a subjective judgment by the clinician as to the "understandability" of the patient's speech. The most common error is to have too low a threshold for disorganization, leading to an overdiagnosis of Schizophrenia. It is unwise to assume that every subtle illogical shift from one topic to another has pathological significance. Latitude should be given to account for variations in style, particularly in the stressful situation of a psychiatric interview. Only speech that is severely disorganized and very difficult to interpret should be considered for a rating of "+". A final caution is that the clinician's unfamiliarity with the patient's dialect or accent or the patient's lack of proficiency in the clinician's language should not be misdiagnosed as disorganized speech.

Grossly disorganized behavior. Two judgments are required here—that the behavior is "disorganized" and that it is severe ("grossly"). Disorganized behavior does not have any apparent goal. Examples of disorganized behavior include wandering around aimlessly and unpredictably shouting at passersby. It is important to exclude behavior that may appear disorganized or bizarre but in fact has a goal (e.g., collecting worthless items from trash dumpsters in response to a delusion that they would provide protection against radiation). In order to justify a rating of "+", the disorganization must be severely impairing to the patient and obvious even to the most casual observer.

Catatonic behavior. These symptoms (item label B22) come from the DSM-5 criteria set (p. 119) for Catatonia Associated With Another Mental Disorder. These catatonia items are almost always coded based on historical information from informants or after a review of prior records, because patients with catatonia are typically unable to provide such information firsthand. Note that the order of the items has been changed from the DSM-5 Catatonia criteria set so that items are grouped together based on how they are assessed: the six items assessed by observation (or by informants, including chart review; e.g., grimacing), followed by the three items assessed during the interview or by informants (e.g., echolalia), followed by the three items assessed during physical examination or by informants (e.g., waxy flexibility).

10.4.4 Ratings of Negative Symptoms (B23–B24)

The main problem with the assessment of negative symptoms is overdiagnosis. Like disorganized speech and grossly disorganized behavior, there is a continuum of severity for each of the negative symptoms, and only the most severe, pervasive, persistent, and impairing forms should warrant a rating of "+". For example, the range of affective expression varies widely in the population and among different cultural groups. Many people are laconic without having negative symptoms. The lack of goal direction meant to be conveyed by the term *avolition* is at the extreme end of a spectrum and should not be confused with lesser and more common difficulties in getting started at things. Furthermore, it is important to ensure that other explanations for the behavior be considered and ruled out before considering the negative symptoms to be "primary" and rating these items "+". The most common confusion in this regard is probably due to the fact that the very medications used to treat psychotic disorders can produce side effects that mimic negative symptoms. For example, many patients taking an antipsychotic medication experience loss of facial expressiveness, reduced speech and movements, dysphoria, and loss of energy. It may be useful to inquire whether presumptive negative symptoms were present before the onset of the neuroleptic treatment, and the potential impact of a reduction or change in medication or the addition of an anticholinergic agent on the symptoms can sometimes be informative. It can also be difficult to distinguish between negative symptoms (avolition and diminished emotional expressiveness) and depressive symptoms (constricted affect, psychomotor retardation, indecisiveness, loss of energy, and loss of pleasure) that not infrequently accompany psychotic disorders. Finally, negative symptoms must be differentiated from behaviors that are secondary to positive symptoms. For example, a patient who is unable to maintain a job because of persecutory delusions would not necessarily be counted as having avolition.

In order to emphasize the importance of not overdiagnosing negative symptoms, the clinician is required to rate each negative symptom twice. The initial rating indicates the apparent presence of the symptom, and if the symptom is present, the second rating confirms that the symptom is in fact *primary* (e.g., a negative symptom of Schizophrenia) rather than *secondary* (e.g., a side effect of medication, a depressive symptom, or the consequence of a positive symptom). Note that use of the terms "primary" and "secondary" in the context of negative symptoms differs in meaning from use of the terms in the context of ruling out a general medical or substance/medication-induced etiology throughout the SCID, although in both cases the terms mean that the symptoms are not in fact due to an identifiable cause.

10.5   Module C.   Differential Diagnosis of Psychotic Disorders

This module helps the clinician to make a differential diagnosis of psychotic disorders based on information obtained in Modules A and B. This module is skipped if there has never been a psychotic symptom. At the beginning of Module C, the clinician is directed to Module D ("Differential Diagnosis of Mood Disorders") to assess psychotic symptoms that occur exclusively during a mood disorder. Module C contains assessments of the following Schizophrenia Spectrum and Other Psychotic Disorders:

- Schizophrenia
- Schizophreniform Disorder
- Schizoaffective Disorder
- Delusional Disorder
- Brief Psychotic Disorder
- Psychotic Disorder Due to Another Medical Condition
- Substance/Medication-Induced Psychotic Disorder
- Other Specified Psychotic Disorder

Structurally, this module differs from Modules A and B in several ways. The goal in Module C is to determine which Schizophrenia Spectrum and Other Psychotic Disorder best accounts for the symptoms rated in Modules A and B, whereas the primary goal in Modules A and B is to collect specific information from the patient (and/or informants) about the clinical presentation in order to determine whether individual criteria are met. Proceeding through Module C is akin to moving down a decision tree for psychotic symptoms, such as in the Delusions Decision Tree in the *DSM-5 Handbook of Differential Diagnosis* (First 2014; pp. 38–43). The main focus of the clinician's efforts is on the consideration of whether the criterion in each box is present or absent. A rating of "YES" is made if the criterion is met and a rating of "NO" applies if the criterion is not met. If the clinician is unable to decide whether or not a criterion has been met because of missing information (e.g., the patient is a poor historian, old charts are unavailable), the clinician always has the option of skipping to item label C22 and making a diagnosis of Other Specified Psychotic Disorder. Because many of these criteria have multiple clauses and involve double negatives, notes are provided at the bottom of many of the criterion item boxes as a quick guide to making the ratings. It is suggested that the clinician review the notes before making a final rating to confirm that the criterion has been correctly interpreted.

For most of the items in Module C, there is no need to ask a question, although for some items additional questions may be required for clarification, especially for those criteria requiring a judgment about the temporal relationships of symptoms. For example, as shown in item label C1 below, although it is possible that the clinician might have sufficient information about the temporal relationship between the mood episodes in Module A and the psychotic symptoms in Module B to rate this item, in most cases it is advantageous to ask the patient this question in order to verify the temporal relationships between the mood and psychotic symptoms.

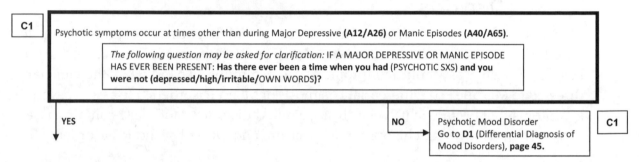

Under typical circumstances, the latter half of Module B and most of Module C is assessed without the need to ask the patient any additional questions. Thus, from the patient's perspective, often the last thing heard aloud until the beginning of Alcohol Use Disorders in Module E is the clinician saying, "Let me stop for a minute while I make a few notes" (between item labels B19 and B20), followed by the clinician flipping through pages and making item ratings while the patient looks on. In order to minimize the patient's waiting time, it is advisable for the clinician to become proficient with this section so it can be done quickly and efficiently. We strongly recommend that novice SCID-5-CV users practice going through Modules C and D using the Homework Cases in Appendix B, "Training Materials," in this User's Guide. We caution against the practice of skipping Module C with the idea that it can be completed later when the patient is no longer present, because additional questions of the patient may be required in order to rate certain criteria.

Note that there are two situations in which the clinician may need to return to Module A to recode items after completing Modules B and C:

1. If the diagnosis of Persistent Depressive Disorder was made in Module A and then a Schizophrenia Spectrum and Other Psychotic Disorder diagnosis is made in Module C, the rating for Criterion F (item label A88) in Persistent Depressive Disorder (i.e., "is not better explained by a persistent…Psychotic Disorder") may need to be recoded; OR

2. Because of the difficulty distinguishing the negative symptoms of Schizophrenia from symptoms of depression, a Major Depressive Episode that has been previously diagnosed in Module A might need to be recoded if a diagnosis of Schizophrenia is later made in Module C. In such cases, the clinician should return to Module A and recode any items as "—" if they are determined to be negative symptoms of Schizophrenia.

10.5.1   R/O Psychotic Mood Disorder (C1)

The hallmark of the diagnoses of Bipolar Disorder With Psychotic Features and Major Depressive Disorder With Psychotic Features is that the psychotic symptoms occur only during mood episodes. Thus, the initial step in the differential diagnosis of mood and psychotic symptoms is to skip out of Module C (Differential Diagnosis of Psychotic Disorders) and continue with Module D (Differential Diagnosis of Mood Disorders) if all the psychotic symptoms are confined to episodes of mood disorder. This initial criterion is not actually part of the criteria set for any DSM-5 disorder but has been included in the SCID-5-CV to allow the clinician to skip past the evaluation of nonmood psychotic disorder if psychotic symptoms are confined to mood episodes.

10.5.2   Ratings for Schizophrenia (C2–C6)

The criteria for Schizophrenia are presented in the SCID in a different order than in DSM-5 to maximize diagnostic efficiency. For example, the clinician immediately skips out of Schizophrenia if the temporal relationship between mood and psychotic symptoms indicates Schizoaffective Disorder or a Depressive or Bipolar Disorder With Psychotic Features. Similarly, Criterion C (duration of at least 6 months) precedes Criterion B (decline in functioning) to allow the clinician to immediately skip out of the assessment of Schizophrenia and continue with Schizophreniform Disorder if the duration is less than 6 months.

Criterion A—Active-phase symptoms.   This criterion defines the active phase of Schizophrenia, which is required at some point during the individual's lifetime for a diagnosis of Schizophrenia to be warranted. Note that in some cases the active-phase symptoms may have been present many years before the interview. This criterion requires that two out of the five listed Criterion A symptoms must have been present for a significant portion of time during a 1-month period (or "less if successfully treated"), one symptom of which must have been delusions, hallucinations, or disorganized speech. The clinician will need to refer to the ratings of the corresponding psychotic symptoms in Module B in order to score Criterion A and must determine both a minimum duration (i.e., was it a significant portion of time during a 1-month period?) and the fact that at least two symptoms have clustered during the same period of time. Note that the inclusion of the phrase "less if successfully treated" acknowledges that clinical judgment is required when applying the duration criterion. For a patient who has been promptly and aggressively treated with antipsychotic medication, if the other aspects of the illness are unequivocally present, the 1-month duration requirement is waived.

Criterion D—Rule out Schizoaffective Disorder. For presentations characterized by a mixture of mood and psychotic symptoms that meet Criterion A for Schizophrenia, the differential diagnosis includes Schizophrenia, Schizoaffective Disorder, and Depressive or Bipolar Disorder With Psychotic Features. As discussed above, the clinician has already been instructed in item label C1 to skip out of Module C if the psychotic symptoms are confined to Depressive and Manic Episodes (indicating that the diagnosis is Depressive or Bipolar Disorder With Psychotic Features), leaving the differential diagnosis to Schizophrenia or Schizoaffective Disorder. Criterion D delineates the admittedly inexact boundary between Schizophrenia and Schizoaffective Disorder—a rating of "YES" on this item indicates that Schizoaffective Disorder has been ruled out, and the clinician continues with Schizophrenia Criterion C (item label C4 on page 38). A "NO" rating for Criterion D indicates that the diagnosis is more likely to be Schizoaffective Disorder and that the interview should resume with item label C9 on page 39.

The two essential aspects of the boundary between Schizophrenia and Schizoaffective Disorder are embodied in the two different parts of Criterion D. The first part operationalizes the requirement in Schizoaffective Disorder that mood episodes occur concurrently with the active-phase symptoms of Schizophrenia (corresponding to Criterion A in Schizoaffective Disorder). If this is not the case, then Schizoaffective Disorder is ruled out on this ground alone and the clinician can continue with Schizophrenia Criterion C (item label C4). Note that the first part of Criterion D is a double negative—we recommend that the clinician follow the instructions laid out in the note below Criterion D in order to prevent making a wrong turn here!

If there is a Major Depressive or Manic Episode occurring concurrently with the psychotic symptoms (suggesting the possibility of Schizoaffective Disorder), the clinician must then evaluate the second half of Criterion D to determine the relationship between the duration of the mood episodes and the total duration of the psychotic disturbance. If the total duration of the mood episodes is less than 50% (i.e., a minority) of the total duration of the psychotic disturbance (including active and residual periods), then this criterion should be rated "YES" and the clinician should continue with the assessment of the remaining criteria for Schizophrenia. If, on the other hand, the total duration of the mood episodes adds up to 50% (or more) of the total duration of the psychotic disturbance, then Criterion D is rated "NO" and the clinician proceeds with the criteria for Schizoaffective Disorder (item label C9, page 39).

Criterion C—Disturbance persists for at least 6 months. The 6-month duration criterion, which differentiates Schizophrenia from Schizophreniform Disorder, is generally only an issue in patients who are having their first psychotic break. Note that the 6-month duration includes any combination of active, prodromal, and residual symptoms. A patient is considered to be in the prodromal or residual phase of Schizophrenia if there are considerable negative symptoms equivalent to those present during the active phase (see Schizophrenia Criterion A5). Alternatively, the patient can be considered to be in the prodromal or residual phase if there are milder versions of the symptoms listed in Schizophrenia Criteria A1–A4. For example, the patient may have overvalued ideas, ideas of reference, or magical thinking with content similar to what, in the active phase, is a delusional conviction, but they have not yet developed frank delusions or they are recovering from a phase of having frank delusions. Similarly, a patient who experiences hallucinations during the active phase may have unusual perceptual experiences in the prodromal or residual periods (e.g., recurrent illusions, perceptions of auras, sensing a force). Disorganized speech that is incoherent during the active phase may be digressive, vague, or overelaborate in the prodromal or residual periods. The patient may continue to act in a peculiar fashion but no longer exhibit grossly disorganized behavior.

Note that the listing of prodromal/residual symptoms in item label C4 (page 38) of the SCID-5-CV has been adapted from the DSM-5 text (p. 101) and the DSM-III-R list of prodromal/residual symptoms (pp. 194–195), which was the last DSM edition to explicitly list prodromal/residual symptoms.

Criterion B—Failure to achieve expected level(s) of functioning.   Areas of functioning include work or school, interpersonal relations, and self-care. Functional impairment resulting from the above symptoms is usually quite evident from the Overview, so this is a question that the clinician will usually not need to ask.

Criterion E—Not due to a GMC and not substance/medication-induced.   This criterion instructs the clinician to consider and rule out a GMC or a substance/medication as an etiological factor. See Section 9, "Differentiating General Medical and Substance/Medication Etiologies From Primary Disorders," in this User's Guide for a discussion of how to rate this criterion. If the clinician decides that the diagnosis is Psychotic Disorder Due to Another Medical Condition or Substance/Medication-Induced Psychotic Disorder, that diagnosis should be recorded in the Diagnostic Summary Score Sheet under Schizophrenia Spectrum and Other Psychotic Disorders. Note that the presence of certain psychotic symptoms (e.g., hallucinations in modalities other than auditory) or an atypical course (e.g., first onset of psychotic symptoms after age 60) strongly suggests the possibility of a GMC or substance/medication etiology.

If the patient has had a primary psychotic disorder but also has psychotic symptoms that are due to a GMC or a substance/medication, both the primary psychotic disorder and Psychotic Disorder Due to Another Medical Condition or Substance/Medication-Induced Psychotic Disorder can be diagnosed by going through Module C more than once (i.e., one time for the primary psychotic symptoms and a second time for the "organic psychosis"). For this reason, the "NO" arrow coming down from item label C6 points to a box instructing the clinician to go back to item label C2 (page 37) and go through Module C again after making the diagnosis of Psychotic Disorder Due to Another Medical Condition or Substance/Medication-Induced Psychotic Disorder if there is evidence that the patient has also had psychotic symptoms at other times (i.e., when not suffering from a GMC and/or when not using substances/medications).

10.5.3   Ratings for Schizophreniform Disorder (C7–C8)

The SCID-5-CV resumes at this point if Criteria A and D of Schizophrenia are present (i.e., active-phase symptoms for at least 1 month, and Schizoaffective Disorder has been ruled out) *but* Criterion C is not true (i.e., total duration is NOT greater than 6 months).

Criterion B—Duration of at least 1 month but less than 6 months.   It is important to ensure that the psychotic symptoms have lasted for at least 1 month in the assessment of Schizophreniform Disorder, because it is possible to reach this point in the SCID-5-CV when psychotic symptoms have lasted for less than 1 month (e.g., delusions and hallucinations that remitted after 2 weeks due to successful treatment with neuroleptics). For psychotic symptoms lasting less than 1 month, the SCID-5-CV skips to the assessment of Brief Psychotic Disorder, item label C19 on page 41.

Criterion D—Not due to a GMC and not substance/medication-induced.   This criterion instructs the clinician to consider and rule out a GMC or a substance/medication as an etiological factor. See Section 9, "Differentiating General Medical and Substance/ Medication Etiologies From Primary Disorders," in this User's Guide for a discussion of how to rate this criterion. If the clinician decides that the diagnosis is Psychotic Disorder Due to Another Medical Condition or Substance/Medication-Induced Psychotic Disorder, that diagnosis should be recorded in the Diagnostic Summary Score Sheet under Schizophrenia Spectrum and Other Psychotic Disorders. Note that the presence of certain psychotic symptoms (e.g., hallucinations in modalities other than auditory) or an atypical course (e.g., first onset of psychotic symptoms after age 60) strongly suggests the possibility of a GMC or substance/medication etiology.

   If the patient has had a primary psychotic disorder but also has psychotic symptoms that are due to a GMC or a substance/medication, both the primary psychotic disorder and Psychotic Disorder Due to Another Medical Condition or Substance/Medication-Induced Psychotic Disorder can be diagnosed by going through Module C more than once (i.e., one time for the primary psychotic symptoms and a second time for the "organic psychosis"). For this reason, the "NO" arrow coming down from item label C8 points to a box instructing the clinician to go back to item label C2 (page 37) and go through Module C again after making the diagnosis of Psychotic Disorder Due to Another Medical Condition or Substance/Medication-Induced Psychotic Disorder if there is evidence that the patient has also had psychotic symptoms at other times (i.e., when not suffering from a GMC and/or when not using substances/medications).

10.5.4   Ratings for Schizoaffective Disorder (C9–C12)

The SCID-5-CV interview picks up at this point if the following apply:

1. Criterion A for Schizophrenia (item label C2) is rated "YES" (i.e., active-phase symptoms for at least 1 month); and
2. Both Criterion D1 and Criterion D2 for Schizophrenia are absent; thus, item label C3 is rated "NO" (i.e., there is a period of overlap between mood episodes and psy-

chotic symptoms AND the total duration of the mood episodes is 50% or more of the total duration of the disturbance).

Criterion A—Duration.   It is assumed that the minimum duration of a Major Depressive Episode or Manic Episode applies, although no minimum duration is explicitly noted in this criterion. Therefore the overlapping period of mood and psychotic symptoms must be at least 2 weeks for a Major Depressive Episode or 1 week for a Manic Episode. Actual durations of mood episodes in Schizoaffective Disorder are usually much longer, comprising months or even years.

It can be a clinical challenge to sort out the degree to which a particular symptom is attributable to a mood episode, Criterion A of Schizophrenia, a medication side effect, or some combination of the three. For example, depressive symptoms can be difficult to distinguish from negative symptoms or antipsychotic medication side effects, and it can be difficult to determine whether disorganized, excited behavior is part of Criterion A of Schizophrenia or characteristic of a Manic Episode. For this reason, Major Depressive Episodes occurring as part of Schizoaffective Disorder must, by definition, be characterized by the presence of depressed mood and not only by its alternative symptom, decreased interest or pleasure in activities (which can be indistinguishable from anhedonia, a typical negative symptom).

Criterion B—Delusions or hallucinations in the absence of mood episodes.   This criterion ensures that the delusions or hallucinations have lasted for at least 2 weeks in the absence of a Manic or Major Depressive Episode. Criterion B theoretically serves to distinguish Schizoaffective Disorder from Mood Disorder With Psychotic Features, because in prototypical Bipolar or Major Depressive Disorder With Psychotic Features, the psychotic symptoms are completely confined to the Mood Disorder episodes. However, given that the clinician already asked whether all of the patient's psychotic symptoms were confined to Manic or Major Depressive Episodes (item label C1), a "NO" rating for Criterion B (item label C10) indicates that any psychotic symptoms that have occurred outside of the mood episodes have lasted less than 2 weeks—thus ruling out both Mood Disorder With Psychotic Features and Schizoaffective Disorder. Such cases (i.e., those rated "NO") are diagnosed as Other Specified Psychotic Disorder.

Criterion C—Mood episodes present for majority of the time.   This item is the inverse of Criterion D2 for Schizophrenia (i.e., "if mood episodes have occurred during active-phase symptoms, they have been present for a minority [i.e., less than 50%] of the total duration of the active and residual periods of the illness") and thus requires that the total duration of mood episodes has been 50% or more of the total duration of the disturbance. Theoretically, it should not be possible to make a rating other than "YES," because the clinician would not ordinarily reach this point in the SCID-5-CV unless Criterion D2 in Schizophrenia was rated "NO." If for some reason this was not the case, then the diagnosis would be Other Specified Psychotic Disorder.

Criterion D—Not due to a GMC and not substance/medication-induced. This criterion instructs the clinician to consider and rule out a GMC or a substance/medication as an etiological factor. See Section 9, "Differentiating General Medical and Substance/Medication Etiologies From Primary Disorders," in this User's Guide for a discussion of how to rate this criterion. If the clinician decides that the diagnosis is Psychotic Disorder Due to Another Medical Condition or Substance/Medication-Induced Psychotic Disorder, that diagnosis should be recorded in the Diagnostic Summary Score Sheet under Schizophrenia Spectrum and Other Psychotic Disorders. Note that the presence of certain psychotic symptoms (e.g., hallucinations in modalities other than auditory) or an atypical course (e.g., first onset of psychotic symptoms after age 60) strongly suggests the possibility of a GMC or substance/medication etiology.

If the patient has had a primary psychotic disorder but also has psychotic symptoms that are due to a GMC or a substance/medication, both the primary psychotic disorder and Psychotic Disorder Due to Another Medical Condition or Substance/Medication-Induced Psychotic Disorder can be diagnosed by going through Module C more than once (i.e., one time for the primary psychotic symptoms and a second time for the "organic psychosis"). For this reason, the "NO" arrow coming down from item label C12 points to a box instructing the clinician to go back to item C2 (page 37) and go through Module C again after making the diagnosis of Psychotic Disorder Due to Another Medical Condition or Substance/Medication-Induced Psychotic Disorder if there is evidence that the patient has also had psychotic symptoms at other times (i.e., when not suffering from a GMC and/or when not using substances/medications).

10.5.5   Ratings for Delusional Disorder (C13–C18)

The SCID-5-CV interview resumes at this point if Criterion A for Schizophrenia is not met (as assessed in item label C2; i.e., two or more of the five active-phase symptoms have never been present during the same 1-month period)—thus ruling out Schizophrenia, Schizophreniform Disorder, and Schizoaffective Disorder.

Criterion A—Delusions for 1 month or longer. Delusional Disorder requires at least 1 month of delusions that occur generally in the absence of other psychotic symptoms. If the patient's distorted beliefs, however, are restricted to his or her appearance or the feared consequences of not performing a compulsion, the clinician is asked to consider whether the delusions are better explained by a diagnosis of Body Dysmorphic Disorder or Obsessive-Compulsive Disorder, With Absent Insight/Delusional Beliefs. If so, the clinician should then skip out of the assessment of Delusional Disorder and continue with item label D1 (Differential Diagnosis of Mood Disorders).

Criterion B—Criterion A for Schizophrenia never met. There should never have been a time lasting a month or more during which active-phase symptoms of Schizophrenia have been concurrent with the delusions. An exception to this requirement is made for chronic olfactory or tactile hallucinations that are thematically related to the delusion (e.g., a patient having the perception of emitting a foul body odor related to the delusion that neighbors are avoiding him).

Criterion C—No other symptoms or impairment.   In contrast to Schizophrenia, an individual with Delusional Disorder will often appear to have no mental illness as long as the clinician has not tapped into the delusional system.

Criterion D—Mood episodes are brief relative to delusional disturbance.   Analogous to Criterion D in Schizophrenia, this criterion guides the differential diagnosis for individuals with mood episodes and long-standing delusions. If the patient has had mood episodes that have been relatively brief compared with the total duration of the delusions, then the diagnosis is consistent with Delusional Disorder, and the clinician is instructed to code "YES" and continue with the evaluation of the remaining Delusional Disorder criteria. For example, persistent and prominent delusions for many years with only occasional and relatively brief mood episodes would be diagnosed as Delusional Disorder. If the mood episodes are not brief compared with the duration of the delusions, the differential diagnosis is between either 1) Mood Disorder With Psychotic Features, if the delusions occur only during mood episodes; or 2) Other Specified Psychotic Disorder, for presentations in which the mood episodes are not brief, yet there are periods of time when the patient is delusional in the absence of significant mood symptoms. (Schizoaffective Disorder is not one of the differential diagnoses; it requires that the psychotic symptoms meet Criterion A of Schizophrenia, thus requiring psychotic symptoms in addition to the delusions.) Given that Module C began by having the clinician evaluate whether the psychotic symptoms occurred only during mood episodes (in which case the clinician was instructed to skip directly to Module D), the only presentations that remain are delusions with mood episodes that were not brief; thus, a rating of "NO" for Criterion D results in a skip to Other Specified Psychotic Disorder.

Criterion E—Not due to a GMC and not substance/medication-induced or due to another mental disorder.   The first part of this criterion instructs the clinician to consider and rule out a GMC or a substance/medication as an etiological factor. See Section 9, "Differentiating General Medical and Substance/Medication Etiologies From Primary Disorders," in this User's Guide for a discussion of how to rate this criterion. If the clinician decides that the diagnosis is Psychotic Disorder Due to Another Medical Condition or Substance/Medication-Induced Psychotic Disorder, that diagnosis should be recorded in the Diagnostic Summary Score Sheet under Schizophrenia Spectrum and Other Psychotic Disorders. Note that the presence of certain psychotic symptoms (e.g., hallucinations in modalities other than auditory) or an atypical course (e.g., first onset of psychotic symptoms after age 60) strongly suggests the possibility of a GMC or substance/medication etiology.

If the patient has had a primary psychotic disorder but also has psychotic symptoms that are due to a GMC or a substance/medication, both the primary psychotic disorder and Psychotic Disorder Due to Another Medical Condition or Substance/Medication-Induced Psychotic Disorder can be diagnosed by going through Module C more than once (i.e., one time for the primary psychotic symptoms and a second time for the "organic psychosis"). For this reason, the "NO" arrow coming down from item label C17 points to a box instructing the clinician to go back to item label C2 (page 37) and go through Module C again after making the diagnosis of Psychotic Disorder Due to Another Medical Condition or Substance/Medication-Induced Psychotic Disorder if there is evidence that the patient has also had psychotic symptoms at other times (i.e., when not suffering from a GMC and/or when not using substances/medications).

The second part reminds the clinician to not make the diagnosis of Delusional Disorder if the symptoms are better explained by another mental disorder. Delusional forms of OCD and Body Dysmorphic Disorder have already been excluded through the skip instruction that appears at the beginning of the assessment of Delusional Disorder. Note that delusional forms of Illness Anxiety Disorder (e.g., being convinced that one is dying of a brain tumor despite the absence of supportive medical evidence) are included in Delusional Disorder and are not excluded (i.e., there is no With Absent Insight/Delusional Beliefs specifier associated with this disorder).

10.5.6   Ratings for Brief Psychotic Disorder (C19–C21)

This diagnosis applies to psychotic episodes that last at least 1 day, but less than 1 month, and are not part of a mood disorder, any of the more specific psychotic disorders described above, or a Psychotic Disorder Due to Another Medical Condition or a Substance/Medication-Induced Psychotic Disorder.

10.5.7   Ratings for Other Specified Psychotic Disorder (C22–C24)

The paragraph defining this disorder (DSM-5, p. 122) has been converted into a set of three ratings included in the SCID-5-CV. Note that the full name of this residual category is Other Specified Schizophrenia Spectrum and Other Psychotic Disorder in DSM-5 but was simplified as Other Specified Psychotic Disorder for the purposes of the SCID. Moreover, Other Specified Psychotic Disorder combines the DSM-5 categories of Other Specified *and* Unspecified Schizophrenia Spectrum and Other Psychotic Disorders, given that the difference depends entirely on coding and recording issues (i.e., "Other Specified" applies if the clinician chooses to indicate the reason why the presentation did not meet criteria for a specific Schizophrenia Spectrum and Other Psychotic Disorder, and "Unspecified" applies if the clinician chooses *not* to indicate the reason). Thus, the clinician will differentiate between the "Other Specified" and "Unspecified" categories only on the Diagnostic Summary Score Sheet.

Symptoms characteristic of a Schizophrenia Spectrum and Other Psychotic Disorder.   This category is intended for presentations "characteristic" of a Schizophrenia Spectrum and Other Psychotic Disorder that predominate the clinical picture (i.e., abnormalities in one of the five domains that define Schizophrenia Spectrum and Other Psychotic Disorders: delusions, hallucinations, disorganized speech, disorganized or abnormal motor behavior, and negative symptoms).

Symptoms cause clinically significant distress or impairment.   This item clarifies that the category, like all of the Other Specified categories, must meet the basic requirement that the symptoms are sufficiently severe to have a negative impact on the patient's life.

Not due to a GMC and not substance/medication-induced.   This item instructs the clinician to consider and rule out a GMC or a substance/medication as an etiological factor. See Section 9, "Differentiating General Medical and Substance/Medication Etiologies From Primary Disorders," in this User's Guide for a discussion of how to rate this criterion. If the clinician decides that the diagnosis is Psychotic Disorder Due to Another Medical Condition or Substance/Medication-Induced Psychotic Disorder, that diagnosis should be recorded in the Diagnostic Summary Score Sheet under Schizophrenia Spectrum and Other Psychotic Disorders.

10.5.8   Ratings for Chronology of Psychotic Disorders (C25–C30)

After making a diagnosis of one of the Schizophrenia Spectrum and Other Psychotic Disorders, the clinician is directed to this Chronology section to determine whether or not the disorder is current, a decision for which no explicit guidance is provided in DSM-5. Requiring that the full criteria be met for the entire past month, as is done for other disorders in the SCID-5-CV, does not work for the psychotic disorders. Thus, the minimum duration thresholds that are part of the diagnostic criteria for the various Schizophrenia Spectrum and Other Psychotic Disorders do not apply to the determination of whether the disorder is "current." After consultation with the DSM-5 Psychotic Disorders Work Group, the following disorder-specific criteria indicative of active illness have been adopted in the SCID-5-CV:

1. **Schizophrenia** (item label C25)—The disorder is considered to be current if active-phase criteria are met for any duration in the past month.
2. **Schizophreniform Disorder** (item label C26)—The disorder is considered to be current if active-phase criteria are met for any duration in the past month.
3. **Schizoaffective Disorder** (item label C27)—The disorder is considered to be current if EITHER symptoms meeting criteria for a Manic or Major Depressive Episode (except for duration) are concurrent with symptoms meeting Criterion A of Schizophrenia at some point in the past month OR there have been delusions or hallucinations in the absence of a Manic or Major Depressive Episode in the past month.
4. **Delusional Disorder** (item label C28)—The disorder is considered to be current if delusions are present at any time in the past month.
5. **Brief Psychotic Disorder** (item label C29)—The disorder is considered to be current if delusions, hallucinations, or disorganized speech are present at some point in the past month.
6. **Other Specified Psychotic Disorder** (item label C30)—The disorder is considered to be current if there have been psychotic symptoms in the past month.

For each of these disorders, if criteria are met for being "current," a rating of "YES" should be made, indicating that the Schizophrenia Spectrum and Other Psychotic Disorder diagnosis is current, and the "Current" box should be checked in the appropriate row on the Diagnostic Summary Score Sheet. If the current criteria are *not* met, the item should be rated "NO" (indicating a past history of the diagnosis) and the "Past History" box should be checked in the appropriate row on the Diagnostic Summary Score Sheet.

On the Diagnostic Summary Score Sheet, the applicable row for Other Specified/ Unspecified Schizophrenia Spectrum and Other Psychotic Disorder depends on whether the DSM-5 diagnosis is Other Specified Schizophrenia Spectrum and Other Psychotic Disorder *or* Unspecified Schizophrenia Spectrum and Other Psychotic Disorder. The diagnosis should be Other Specified Schizophrenia Spectrum and Other Psychotic Disorder (and the corresponding box on the Diagnostic Summary Score Sheet should be checked) if the clinician chooses to indicate on the Diagnostic Summary Score Sheet in the space provided the reason why the presentation did not meet criteria for a specific Schizophrenia Spectrum and Other Psychotic Disorder. Otherwise, the diagnosis should be Unspecified Schizophrenia Spectrum and Other Psychotic Disorder, and the corresponding box on the Diagnostic Summary Score Sheet should be checked.

10.6   Module D.   Differential Diagnosis of Mood Disorders

Whereas Module A was for rating Major Depressive, Manic, and Hypomanic Episodes, this module is for recording Bipolar I Disorder, Bipolar II Disorder, Other Specified Bipolar Disorder (including Cyclothymic Disorder), Major Depressive Disorder, and Other Specified Depressive Disorder. The clinician should go through this module if EITHER 1) there have been one or more current or past mood episodes (from Module A) and these mood episodes have not all been subsumed as part of a diagnosis of Schizoaffective Disorder (from Module C); OR 2) there have been clinically significant mood symptoms that do not meet the criteria for a mood episode or mood disorder, such as Persistent Depressive Disorder. (The converse of these conditions is expressed in the skip instruction at the beginning of Module D, item label D1 (i.e., "If there have never been any clinically significant mood symptoms or if all mood symptoms are accounted for by a diagnosis of Schizoaffective Disorder," the clinician is instructed to skip to Module E [Substance Use Disorders], item label E1.) As in Module C, the task in Module D is to evaluate whether the specific criteria for mood disorders are met based on information gathered in Modules A, B, and C.

10.6.1   Ratings for Bipolar I Disorder (D2–D3)

Criterion A—At least one Manic Episode.   The minimum requirement for a diagnosis of Bipolar I Disorder is one Manic Episode during the patient's lifetime. Thus, this item is rated "YES" if there has been either a current Manic Episode or a past Manic Episode in Module A.

Criterion B—The occurrence of the mood episodes is not better explained by Schizoaffective Disorder or another psychotic disorder.   If a psychotic disorder has already been diagnosed in Module C, whether or not a comorbid diagnosis of Bipolar I

Disorder is given depends on whether the Manic Episodes occurred *in addition to* Schizoaffective Disorder or another psychotic disorder. Given that the presence of a Manic Episode is included in the definition of Schizoaffective Disorder, Manic Episodes occurring in the context of a diagnosis of Schizoaffective Disorder are considered to be "explained" by the Schizoaffective Disorder and do not count toward a diagnosis of Bipolar I Disorder. The interpretation of "better explained by" as it applies to other psychotic disorders, like Schizophrenia and Delusional Disorder, is less clear. The DSM-IV version of this criterion treated Schizoaffective Disorder and the other psychotic disorders differently, excluding a diagnosis of Bipolar I Disorder if the Manic Episodes were "superimposed on Schizophrenia, Schizophreniform Disorder, Delusional Disorder, or Psychotic Disorder Not Otherwise Specified" (p. 388). This had been interpreted as not counting Manic Episodes toward a diagnosis of Bipolar I Disorder if they occurred during the course of a psychotic disorder, necessitating a diagnosis of Bipolar Disorder Not Otherwise Specified in order to indicate superimposed Manic Episodes. In DSM-5, the use of "better explained by" in place of "superimposed on" (and the absence of any DSM-5 text indicating otherwise) suggests that Manic Episodes occurring during a psychotic disorder other than Schizoaffective Disorder could count toward a diagnosis of Bipolar I Disorder, thus justifying comorbid diagnoses of both the psychotic disorder and Bipolar I Disorder.

Type of current (or most recent) episode.   The evaluation of Bipolar I Disorder concludes with the clinician rating the type of the current episode (or most recent episode, if the Bipolar I Disorder is in remission). The type of episode is used in determining the diagnostic code for Bipolar I Disorder, which is recorded later on the Diagnostic Summary Score Sheet. Four types of episodes can be indicated: Manic, Major Depressive, Hypomanic, and Unspecified. An episode is considered to be "Unspecified" if full criteria except for duration are met for a Manic, Major Depressive, or Hypomanic Episode. Note that if criteria are met simultaneously for both a Manic Episode and a Major Depressive Episode, the current (or most recent) episode is considered to be Manic.

10.6.2   Ratings for Bipolar II Disorder (D4–D7)

Criterion A—At least one Hypomanic Episode and at least one Major Depressive Episode.   The minimum requirement for a diagnosis of Bipolar II Disorder is one Hypomanic Episode and one Major Depressive Episode during the patient's lifetime. Thus, this item is rated "YES" if there has ever been a current or past Major Depressive Episode as well as a current or past Hypomanic Episode in Module A.

Criterion B—Never any Manic Episodes or all Manic Episodes are better explained by a Psychotic Disorder.   Although the Module D skip pattern should prevent the clinician from getting to the evaluation of Bipolar II Disorder if there have ever been any Manic Episodes, this item is retained just to be sure.

Criterion C—The occurrence of the Hypomanic and Major Depressive Episodes is not better explained by Schizoaffective Disorder or another psychotic disorder. If a psychotic disorder has already been diagnosed in Module C, whether or not a co-morbid diagnosis of Bipolar II Disorder is given depends on whether the Hypomanic and Major Depressive Episodes have occurred *in addition to* Schizoaffective Disorder or another psychotic disorder. Given that the presence of a Major Depressive Episode is included in the definition of Schizoaffective Disorder, Major Depressive Episodes occurring in the context of a diagnosis of Schizoaffective Disorder are considered to be "explained" by the Schizoaffective Disorder and do not count toward a diagnosis of Bipolar II Disorder. The interpretation of "better explained by" as it applies to other psychotic disorders, like Schizophrenia and Delusional Disorder, is less clear. The DSM-IV version of this criterion treated Schizoaffective Disorder and the other psychotic disorders differently, excluding a diagnosis of Bipolar II Disorder if the Major Depressive Episodes and Hypomanic Episodes were "superimposed on Schizophrenia, Schizophreniform Disorder, Delusional Disorder, or Psychotic Disorder Not Otherwise Specified" (p. 397). This had been interpreted as not counting Major Depressive Episodes and Hypomanic Episodes toward a diagnosis of Bipolar II Disorder if they occurred during the course of a psychotic disorder, necessitating a diagnosis of Bipolar Disorder Not Otherwise Specified in order to indicate superimposed Hypomanic and Major Depressive Episodes. The use of "better explained by" in place of "superimposed on" (and the absence of any DSM-5 text indicating otherwise) suggests that in DSM-5, Major Depresssive Episodes and Hypomanic Episodes occurring during a psychotic disorder other than Schizoaffective Disorder could count toward a diagnosis of Bipolar II Disorder, thus justifying comorbid diagnoses of both the psychotic disorder and Bipolar II Disorder.

Criterion D—Depression or unpredictability causes distress or impairment. In Bipolar II Disorder, the requisite clinically significant distress or impairment can arise either from the Major Depressive Episodes themselves, which are often quite severe, or from the unpredictability of the alternation between depression and hypomania. The Hypomanic Episodes by themselves do not cause distress or impairment.

10.6.3   Ratings for Other Specified Bipolar Disorder (D8–D10)

If there are symptoms characteristic of a Bipolar and Related Disorder that do not meet criteria for Bipolar I Disorder or Bipolar II Disorder, then Other Specified Bipolar and Related Disorder should be considered. The paragraph defining Other Specified Bipolar and Related Disorder (DSM-5, p. 148) has been converted into a set of three ratings in the SCID-5-CV. Other Specified Bipolar Disorder combines the DSM-5 categories of Other Specified *and* Unspecified Bipolar and Related Disorders, given that the difference depends entirely on coding and recording issues (i.e., "Other Specified" applies if the clinician chooses to indicate the reason why the presentation did not meet criteria for a specific Bipolar and Related Disorder, and "Unspecified" applies if the clinician chooses *not* to indicate the reason). Thus, the clinician will differentiate between the "Other Specified" and "Unspecified" categories only on the Diagnostic Summary Score Sheet. Given that the DSM-5 category Cyclothymic Disorder is not included in the SCID-5-CV, patients whose symptoms meet criteria for Cyclothymic Disorder would be diagnosed as Other Specified Bipolar Disorder in the SCID-5-CV.

Symptoms characteristic of a Bipolar and Related Disorder.   This item indicates that this category is intended for presentations that include periods of prominent elevated, euphoric, or irritable mood that do not meet criteria for one of the Bipolar and Related Disorders (i.e., Bipolar I Disorder or Bipolar II Disorder). Because the DSM-5 category Cyclothymic Disorder is not included in the SCID-5-CV, patients whose symptoms meet criteria for Cyclothymic Disorder would be diagnosed as Other Specified Bipolar Disorder in the SCID-5-CV.

Symptoms cause clinically significant distress or impairment.   This item clarifies that this category, like all of the Other Specified categories, must meet the basic requirement that the symptoms are sufficiently severe to have a negative impact on the patient's life.

Not due to a GMC and not substance/medication-induced.   This item instructs the clinician to consider and rule out a GMC or a substance/medication as an etiological factor for the bipolar and related symptoms, in which case a Bipolar and Related Disorder Due to Another Medical Condition or Substance/Medication-Induced Bipolar and Related Disorder is diagnosed. See Section 9, "Differentiating General Medical and Substance/Medication Etiologies From Primary Disorders," in this User's Guide for a discussion of how to rate this criterion. If the clinician decides that the diagnosis is Bipolar Disorder Due to Another Medical Condition or Substance/Medication-Induced Bipolar Disorder, that diagnosis should be recorded in the Diagnostic Summary Score Sheet.

10.6.4   Ratings for Major Depressive Disorder (D11–D13)

At least one Major Depressive Episode.   The minimum requirement for a diagnosis of Major Depressive Disorder is one Major Depressive Episode during the patient's lifetime. No single criterion specifies this in the DSM-5 Major Depressive Disorder criteria set. The first three criteria in Major Depressive Disorder are identical to Criteria A, B, and C of a Major Depressive Episode and thus have been combined into a single item in the SCID-5-CV.

Criterion D—The occurrence is not better explained by Schizoaffective Disorder or another psychotic disorder.   If a psychotic disorder has already been diagnosed in Module C, whether or not a comorbid diagnosis of Major Depressive Disorder is given depends on whether the Major Depressive Episodes have occurred *in addition to* Schizoaffective Disorder or another psychotic disorder. Given that the presence of a Major Depressive Episode is included in the definition of Schizoaffective Disorder, Major Depressive Episodes occurring in the context of a diagnosis of Schizoaffective

Disorder are considered to be "explained" by the Schizoaffective Disorder and do not count toward a diagnosis of Major Depressive Disorder. The interpretation of "better explained by" as it applies to other psychotic disorders, like Schizophrenia and Delusional Disorder, is less clear. The DSM-IV version of this criterion treated Schizoaffective Disorder and the other psychotic disorders differently, excluding a diagnosis of Major Depressive Disorder if the Major Depressive Episodes were "superimposed on Schizophrenia, Schizophreniform Disorder, Delusional Disorder, or Psychotic Disorder Not Otherwise Specified." This had been interpreted as not counting Major Depressive Episodes toward a diagnosis of Major Depressive Disorder if they occurred during the course of a psychotic disorder, necessitating a diagnosis of Depressive Disorder Not Otherwise Specified in order to indicate superimposed Major Depressive Episodes. In DSM-5, the use of "better explained by" in place of "superimposed on" (and the absence of any DSM-5 text indicating otherwise) suggests that Major Depressive Episodes occurring during a psychotic disorder other than Schizoaffective Disorder could count toward a diagnosis of Major Depressive Disorder, thus justifying comorbid diagnoses of both the psychotic disorder and Major Depressive Disorder.

Criterion E—Never any Manic or Hypomanic Episodes.   Although the Module D skip pattern should prevent the clinician from getting to the assessment of Major Depressive Disorder (item label D11) if there have been any Manic or Hypomanic Episodes, this item is retained just to be sure.

Single Episode or Recurrent Episodes.   The evaluation of Major Depressive Disorder concludes with the clinician rating whether a single episode or recurrent episodes occur. The type of episode is used in determining the diagnostic code for Major Depressive Disorder, which is recorded later on the Diagnostic Summary Score Sheet. Note that in order for Major Depressive Disorder to be considered recurrent, the clinician needs only to determine that there was a period lasting at least 2 months in which the depressive symptomatology consistently fell below the five-symptom threshold for a Major Depressive Episode (i.e., a partial remission); a 2-month period of full remission is not required to identify a "recurrence."

10.6.5   Ratings for Other Specified Depressive Disorder (D14–D16)

Other Specified Depressive Disorder should be considered if there are symptoms characteristic of a depressive disorder that do not meet criteria for another depressive disorder or for Adjustment Disorder. The paragraph defining this disorder (DSM-5, p. 183) has been converted into a set of three ratings included in the SCID-5-CV. Other Specified Depressive Disorder combines the DSM-5 categories of Other Specified *and* Unspecified Depressive Disorders, given that the difference depends entirely on coding and recording issues (i.e., "Other Specified" applies if the clinician chooses to indicate the reason why the presentation did not meet criteria for a specific depressive disorder, and "Unspecified" applies if the clinician chooses *not* to indicate the reason). Thus, the clinician will differentiate between the "Other Specified" and "Unspecified" categories only on the Diagnostic Summary Score Sheet.

Symptoms characteristic of a depressive disorder. This item indicates that this category is intended for presentations that include periods of prominent depressed mood or loss of interest or pleasure that do not meet the full criteria for Major Depressive Disorder, Persistent Depressive Disorder, Premenstrual Dysphoric Disorder, or Adjustment Disorder With Depressed Mood or Adjustment Disorder With Mixed Anxiety and Depressed Mood. Note that the clause excluding Adjustment Disorder With Depressed Mood and Adjustment Disorder With Mixed Anxiety and Depressed Mood was mistakenly left out of DSM-5 and has been restored here in the SCID-5-CV. Given that Adjustment Disorder has not yet been diagnosed at this point, the clinician may need to return here and revise this rating if criteria are later met for Adjustment Disorder With Depressed Mood or Adjustment Disorder With Mixed Anxiety and Depressed Mood.

Symptoms cause clinically significant distress or impairment. This item clarifies that this category, like all of the Other Specified categories, must meet the basic requirement that the symptoms are sufficiently severe to have a negative impact on the patient's life.

Not due to a GMC and not substance/medication-induced. This item instructs the clinician to consider and rule out a GMC or a substance/medication as an etiological factor for the depressive symptoms, in which case a Depressive Disorder Due to Another Medical Condition or Substance/Medication-Induced Depressive Disorder is diagnosed. See Section 9, "Differentiating General Medical and Substance/Medication Etiologies From Primary Disorders," in this User's Guide for a discussion of how to rate this criterion. If the clinician decides that the diagnosis is Depressive Disorder Due to Another Medical Condition or Substance/Medication-Induced Depressive Disorder, that diagnosis should be recorded in the Diagnostic Summary Score Sheet under Depressive Disorders.

10.6.6   Ratings for Chronology of Bipolar I and Bipolar II Disorder (D17–D23)

The clinician is taken to this Chronology section after making a diagnosis of Bipolar I Disorder, Bipolar II Disorder, or Other Specified Bipolar Disorder. The first step is for the clinician to select the appropriate item, based on both the diagnosis and the type of current (or most recent) episode, and rate whether the criteria have been met during the past month, as follows:

Bipolar I Disorder. *Current or most recent Manic Episode (item label D17).* If symptomatic criteria are met for a Manic Episode during the past month, the clinician should make a rating of "YES" in item label D17, indicating that Bipolar I Disorder is current. Note that at least the entire minimum required duration (i.e., 1 week for the Manic Episode) should have occurred within the past 4 weeks to be considered current. The clinician should next follow the arrow down to the box where the diagnosis is selected based on the current severity (Mild, Moderate, Severe) and presence of psychotic symptoms, and then check the appropriate "Current" box in the Diagnostic Summary Score Sheet. If symptomatic criteria are not met in the past month, item label D17 should be rated "NO," and the clinician should next follow the arrow down and to the left, to the box where the diagnosis is selected based on the degree of remission (In Partial Remission, In Full Remission). A check should then be placed in the appropriate "Past History" box in the Diagnostic Summary Score Sheet.

Current or most recent Major Depressive Episode (item label D18). If symptomatic criteria are met for a Major Depressive Episode during the past month, the clinician should make a rating of "YES" in item label D18, indicating that the Bipolar I Disorder is current. Note that at least the entire minimum required duration (i.e., 2 weeks for the Major Depressive Episode) should have occurred within the past 4 weeks to be considered current. The clinician should next follow the arrow down to the box where the diagnosis is selected based on the current severity (Mild, Moderate, Severe) and presence of psychotic symptoms, and then check the appropriate "Current" box in the Diagnostic Summary Score Sheet. If symptomatic criteria are not met in the past month, item label D18 should be rated "NO," and the clinician should next follow the arrow down and to the left, to the box where the diagnosis is selected based on the degree of remission (In Partial Remission, In Full Remission). A check should then be placed in the appropriate "Past History" box in the Diagnostic Summary Score Sheet.

Note that if full criteria have been simultaneously met for a Manic Episode, the patient is considered to have a current Manic Episode, With Mixed Features, which should be rated "YES" in item label D17; the Major Depressive Episode rating for item label D18 would be "NO." This diagnostic approach follows DSM-5 Criterion C for the With Mixed Features specifier:

> For individuals whose symptoms meet full episode criteria for both mania and depression simultaneously, the diagnosis should be manic episode, with mixed features, due to the marked impairment and clinical severity of full mania. (p. 150)

Because the SCID-5-CV includes only those specifiers that can be coded, there is not a rating for the With Mixed Features specifier for current Manic Episode as this specifier has no diagnostic code.

Current or most recent Hypomanic Episode (item label D19). If symptomatic criteria are met for a Hypomanic Episode during the past month, the clinician should make a rating of "YES" in item label D19, indicating that the Bipolar I Disorder is current. Note that at least the entire minimum required duration (i.e., 4 days for the Hypomanic Episode) should have occurred within the past 4 weeks to be considered current. The clinician should next follow the arrow down to the box where the diagnosis is selected and then check the "Current" box in the Diagnostic Summary Score Sheet. If symptomatic criteria are not met in the past month, item label D19 should be rated "NO," and the clinician should next follow the arrow down and to the left, to the box where the diagnosis is selected based on the degree of remission (In Partial Remission,

In Full Remission). A check should then be placed in the appropriate "Past History" box in the Diagnostic Summary Score Sheet.

Current or most recent Unspecified Episode (item label D20). If symptomatic criteria are met during the past month for a Manic, Hypomanic, or Major Depressive Episode except for duration, the clinician should make a rating of "YES" in item label D20, indicating that the Bipolar I Disorder is current. The clinician should next follow the arrow down to the box where the diagnosis is selected and then check the "Current" box in the Diagnostic Summary Score Sheet. If symptomatic criteria for a Manic, Hypomanic, or Major Depressive Episode are below threshold in the past month (and the most recent episode met severity but not duration criteria for a Manic, Hypomanic, or Major Depressive Episode), item label D20 should be rated "NO," and the clinician should next follow the arrow down to the box where the diagnosis is selected. A check should then be placed in the "Past History" box in the Diagnostic Summary Score Sheet.

Bipolar II Disorder. *Current or most recent Hypomanic Episode (item label D21).* If symptomatic criteria are met for a Hypomanic Episode during the past month, the clinician should make a rating of "YES" in item label D21, indicating that the Bipolar II Disorder is current. Note that at least the entire minimum required duration (i.e., 4 days for the Hypomanic Episode) should have occurred within the past 4 weeks to be considered current. The clinician should next follow the arrow down to the box where the diagnosis is selected and then check the "Current" box in the Diagnostic Summary Score Sheet. If symptomatic criteria are not met in the past month, item label D21 should be rated "NO," and the clinician should next follow the arrow down and to the left, to the box where the diagnosis is selected based on the degree of remission (In Partial Remission, In Full Remission). A check should then be placed in the appropriate "Past History" box in the Diagnostic Summary Score Sheet.

Current or most recent Major Depressive Episode (item label D22). If symptomatic criteria are met for a Major Depressive Episode during the past month, the clinician should make a rating of "YES" in item label D22, indicating that the Bipolar II Disorder is current. Note that at least the entire minimum required duration (i.e., 2 weeks for the Major Depressive Episode) should have occurred within the past 4 weeks to be considered current. The clinician should next follow the arrow down to the box where the diagnosis is selected based on the current severity (Mild, Moderate, Severe) and presence of psychotic symptoms and then check the appropriate "Current" box in the Diagnostic Summary Score Sheet. If symptomatic criteria are not met in the past month, item label D22 should be rated "NO," and the clinician should next follow the arrow down and to the left, to the box where the diagnosis is selected based on the degree of remission (In Partial Remission, In Full Remission). A check should then be placed in the appropriate "Past History" box in the Diagnostic Summary Score Sheet.

Other Specified Bipolar Disorder (item label D23). If there are symptoms characteristic of a Bipolar and Related Disorder that do not meet criteria for a specific Bipolar and

Related Disorder and that cause clinically significant distress or impairment in the past month, the clinician should make a rating of "YES" in item label D23, indicating that the Other Specified (or Unspecified) Bipolar and Related Disorder is current, and then check the "Current" box in the Diagnostic Summary Score Sheet. If there are no bipolar symptoms in the past month, item label D23 should be rated "NO," and a check should then be placed in the "Past History" box in the Diagnostic Summary Score Sheet.

As noted on the Diagnostic Summary Score Sheet, a coding exception applies to Other Specified Bipolar Disorder. Presentations that meet criteria for Cyclothymic Disorder (which is included in the SCID-5-RV but not the SCID-5-CV) are to be assigned the diagnostic code F34.0 for Cyclothymic Disorder instead of F31.89, the diagnostic code for Other Specified Bipolar Disorder.

10.6.7   Ratings for Chronology of Major Depressive Disorder (D24–D25)

The clinician is taken to this Chronology section after making a diagnosis of Major Depressive Disorder or Other Specified Depressive Disorder. The first step is for the clinician to select the appropriate item based on the diagnosis, as follows:

Major Depressive Disorder (item label D24).   If symptomatic criteria are met for a Major Depressive Episode during the past month, the clinician should make a rating of "YES" in item label D24, indicating that the Major Depressive Disorder is current. Note that at least the entire minimum required duration (i.e., 2 weeks for the Major Depressive Episode) should have occurred within the past month to be considered current. The clinician should next follow the arrow down to the box where the diagnosis is selected based on the number of episodes (Single or Recurrent), current severity (Mild, Moderate, Severe), and presence of psychotic symptoms, and then check the appropriate "Current" box in the Diagnostic Summary Score Sheet. If symptomatic criteria are not met in the past month, item label D24 should be rated "NO," and the clinician should next follow the arrow down and to the left, to the box where the diagnosis is selected based on the number of past episodes and the degree of remission (In Partial Remission, In Full Remission). A check should then be placed in the appropriate "Past History" box in the Diagnostic Summary Score Sheet.

Other Specified Depressive Disorder (item label D25).   If there are depressive symptoms causing clinically significant distress or impairment in the past month, the clinician should make a rating of "YES" in item label D25, indicating that the Other Specified (or Unspecified) Depressive Disorder is current, and then check the "Current" box in the Diagnostic Summary Score Sheet. If there are no depressive symptoms in the past month, item label D25 should be rated "NO," and a check should then be placed in the "Past History" box in the Diagnostic Summary Score Sheet.

10.7   Module E.   Substance Use Disorders

This module contains ratings for the Substance Use Disorders, which cover problems caused by the patient's pattern of substance use. The SCID separates the evaluation of

Alcohol Use Disorder from the other Substance Use Disorders because alcohol is legal, alcohol is more widely used than other substances, and most users do not have problems with it. Psychiatric symptoms (e.g., psychosis, depression, anxiety) related to the direct effects of a substance/medication on the central nervous system are diagnosed as Substance/Medication-Induced Mental Disorders, and these diagnoses are located throughout the SCID-5-CV according to the type of symptom presentation (i.e., Substance/Medication-Induced Depressive Disorder and Substance/Medication-Induced Bipolar and Related Disorder in Modules A and D, Substance/Medication-Induced Psychotic Disorder in Module C, Substance/Medication-Induced Anxiety Disorder in Module F, and Substance/Medication-Induced Obsessive-Compulsive and Related Disorder in Module G).

10.7.1   Ratings for Past-12-Month Alcohol Use Disorder (E1–E13)

Because the last section of the Overview ("Other Current Problems") included two questions regarding current alcohol use (i.e., "In the past month, how much have you been drinking?" "When you drink, who are you usually with? (Are you usually alone or out with other people?)"), the clinician should already have a rough idea of the patient's current alcohol use history when starting the Alcohol Use Disorder section. Thus, with the answers to these Overview questions as background, the clinician starts the Past-12-Month Alcohol Use Disorder evaluation by deciding whether it makes sense to completely skip over the evaluation because of the lack of any evidence suggesting the possibility of an Alcohol Use Disorder in the past 12 months. To make this determination, the clinician begins this section by asking the patient to describe his or her drinking habits. If the patient credibly denies using any alcohol in the past 12 months, then the clinician should skip to the assessment of Nonalcohol Substance Use Disorder in item label E14 on page 56.

If the patient reports having used alcohol in the past 12 months, the clinician follows up with a question to determine whether the patient's past-12-month alcohol use exceeds a minimum threshold (i.e., having drunk alcohol at least six times in the past 12 months), below which an Alcohol Use Disorder is unlikely to have occurred. Note that this question is not inquiring about the number of drinks in the past year, but the number of <u>times</u> (i.e., "drinking events") that the patient has used alcohol. On the low end, such a drinking event could consist of only one drink (e.g., having a glass of wine at dinner or at a bar with friends) but on the extreme end could consist of a night of binge drinking at a college fraternity party during which many drinks are consumed. If the patient's reported use is credibly below the threshold of six times in a year, then the clinician is allowed to skip to the evaluation of Nonalcohol Substance Use Disorder, starting with item label E14 on page 56. The standard SCID-5-CV rule regarding skip-outs applies here in particular: when in doubt, do not skip out!

Alcohol (and other Substance) Use Disorders are characterized by a problematic pattern of alcohol or substance use, leading to clinically significant impairment or distress, as indicated by 2 or more of the following 11 criteria occurring within a 12-month period. The examples in brackets were included with many of these criterion items in

DSM-IV but were removed from DSM-5; they have been added back into the SCID-5-CV to assist the clinician in making reliable ratings.

Criterion A1—Larger amounts/longer periods than intended.   The intent of this item is to capture the patient's failed attempts to put some limits on his or her drinking (e.g., "I'll just have a few beers and then go home"; "I'll stop at the bar for only half an hour"). Note that the breaking of these self-imposed limits (e.g., the patient ends up drinking a couple of six-packs or stays at the bar for several hours) must occur OFTEN in order to be coded "+". There is something of a paradox inherent in the evaluation of this item (and Criterion A2 as well). For this criterion to apply, the patient must have developed enough insight about having a drinking problem (or wanting to avoid developing a drinking problem) to want to control his or her drinking. It is therefore not possible to rate this item as "+" in someone who has a very heavy pattern of use but denies any need or desire to control or cut down use.

Criterion A2—Persistent desire or failed efforts to cut down/control alcohol use. This item is rated "+" under two circumstances. First, if the patient has had a persistent desire to stop, cut down, or control his or her drinking, presumably because of self-awareness that it has been problematic in some way, a rating of "+" would apply. Although DSM-5 leaves the definition of "persistent" up to clinical judgment, a period lasting at least 1 month in which the person's desire to cut back or control drinking occurred for most of the time would be a reasonable minimum duration to count as "persistent." Second, in cases in which the patient does not have a persistent desire to cut down or control drinking but nonetheless has tried unsuccessfully to cut down or control drinking (e.g., in response to repeated demands from family members), a rating of "+" would also apply. Note that for an effort to cut down or control drinking to be considered "successful" (and justify a rating of "—"), the period of controlled or diminished use must have lasted for an extended period of time (e.g., months or years).

Criterion A3—Great deal of time spent on alcohol use.   This item covers the various ways in which drinking may become a central focus of the patient's life: time spent obtaining alcohol, time spent drinking and being intoxicated, and time spent recovering from its effects. Reasonable people may disagree about what constitutes "a great deal of time." As a rule of thumb, two evenings a week spent drinking is not "a great deal of time" and would justify a rating of "—"; most evenings a week with next-day hangovers would justify a rating of "+".

Criterion A4—Craving.   This item is rated "+" if there has been a strong urge or desire to use alcohol when not drinking. The intensity threshold for craving should be such that the craving has some negative impact on the patient. For example, the urge to drink might be so strong that the patient has trouble thinking about anything else, or it results in significant discomfort or greatly weakens the patient's resolve to cut back on or quit drinking alcohol. In some patients, the urge to drink is associated with specific cues, like going into a bar or running into a drinking buddy on the street. In order to explore this possibility, the follow-up question asks whether the craving is associated with certain situations.

Criterion A5—Failure to fulfill obligations at work, school, or home.   A rating of "+" for this item requires specific evidence that the effects of the alcohol use (i.e., intoxication, withdrawal, or hangover) resulted in the patient's failure to fulfill a major role obligation on at least two occasions. The accompanying examples illustrate the wide range of the types of activities that may be affected: repeated absences from work or poor work performance; absences, suspensions, or expulsions from school; and neglect of children or household responsibilities. Simply being intoxicated while at work, school, or taking care of children without apparent impairment is not sufficient to justify a rating of "+"; there must be some evidence that the effects of alcohol significantly and recurrently interfered with functioning in one of these domains.

Criterion A6—Continued use despite recurrent interpersonal problems as a result of alcohol use.   Like Criterion A5, Criterion A6 reflects social or interpersonal problems that are caused by the effects of drinking, such as marital strain caused by arguments or physical fights that occur during periods of intoxication. Unlike Criterion A5, a rating of "+" for Criterion A6 requires that the patient continue to use alcohol despite these problems. This item may be difficult to evaluate when the interpersonal conflict is possibly attributable to an underlying relational problem rather than to the patient's substance use. For example, arguments about occasional nonproblematic drinking that are initiated by a spouse who is against any drinking at all would not warrant a rating of "+".

Criterion A7—Important activities given up at work, school, or home so that time can be spent on alcohol use.   The prototypical patient whose alcohol use meets this criterion is a "street-corner alcoholic" who has essentially given up all activities except those associated with drinking. However, Criterion A7 may also apply, for example, to an amateur athlete who has stopped sports activities because of drinking or to a person who has stopped seeing all her friends so she can stay home and drink.

Criterion A8—Recurrent use in physically hazardous situations.   A common error in rating this item is to be overinclusive and assume that any level of alcohol use in a situation that requires alertness would qualify. The item should be rated "+" only if the alcohol use caused sufficient impairment in coordination or cognition to create a physically hazardous condition (e.g., driving or hunting while intoxicated). To facilitate a proper inquiry, the first question simply establishes that the patient has drunk alcohol before engaging in an activity that requires coordination and concentration. If the patient acknowledges such use, the follow-up question then establishes whether the patient was in fact impaired to a degree that someone could have been injured as a result of the impaired coordination or concentration. Clinical judgment is necessary when interpreting the diagnostic significance of the patient's answers, balancing variability in how much a given individual may be impacted by a given amount of alcohol due to tolerance with patients' tendencies to minimize the impact of alcohol on their coordination and cognition. If a patient acknowledges consuming a great deal of alcohol in a short period of time and yet denies any impact on his or her functioning as a result, the clinician might be justified in "overriding" the patient's negative response and concluding that the patient was in fact impaired, depending on the amount consumed and the person's level of tolerance.

Although getting drunk and walking home through a dangerous neighborhood or having unprotected sex with someone one doesn't know very well while intoxicated is certainly risky, neither would warrant a rating of "+"; the intent of the item is to rate behavior that puts the patient or others in immediate danger because his or her coordination or cognition is impaired by drinking.

Criterion A9—Continued use despite knowledge that physical or psychological problems are caused or made worse by the alcohol.   Like Criterion A6, Criterion A9 is meant to tap a pattern of compulsive alcohol use and does not refer merely to the adverse physical or psychological consequences of drinking. Consequently, for the clinician to rate this item "+", the patient must first acknowledge understanding that the physical or psychological problems that he or she is experiencing are caused by drinking and that despite this knowledge, he or she has continued to drink. Examples of physical problems include cirrhosis or esophageal bleeding due to excessive drinking; examples of psychological problems are "blackouts" (memory loss for events that occurred while intoxicated), alcohol-induced depression, or rebound anxiety the day after a heavy drinking episode. The most frequent noxious physical effect of alcohol is a hangover. When hangovers are severe and frequent and the patient still continues to drink regularly, a rating of "+" is justified.

Criterion A10—Tolerance.   Tolerance is the need for a person to drink greater amounts of alcohol to get the same effect as when that person first started drinking. Although Criterion A10 requires the need for "markedly increased amounts," how much this needs to be is left up to clinical judgment. The DSM-III-R version of the tolerance criterion specified at least a 50% increase, but this requirement was dropped from DSM-IV because it was felt to be pseudoprecise. Any adult who drinks regularly has somewhat more tolerance than when they were normal adolescents experimenting with alcohol. This item is intended to capture those whose tolerance has increased markedly (e.g., "I used to get drunk on three beers. Now I can drink two six-packs and not get drunk").

Criterion A11—Withdrawal.   Withdrawal is indicated by the development of the characteristic alcohol withdrawal syndrome shortly after stopping or decreasing the amount of alcohol. In some cases, the individual never allows the withdrawal syndrome to develop because he or she starts drinking or taking a sedative in anticipation of the onset of withdrawal symptoms, as noted in part (b) of this criterion. For this reason, if the patient denies having had withdrawal symptoms, the clinician asks whether or not the patient has ever started the day with a drink or else drank or took some other medication to avoid getting sick from withdrawal. Note that for part (a) of this criterion, at least two symptoms must develop within several hours to a few days after the cessation (or reduction in) alcohol use. Two or more of the symptoms do not necessarily need to occur at the same time. As the criterion suggests, the course of development of withdrawal symptoms varies according to the symptom, the typical amount of alcohol consumed, and individual differences.

Meeting Criterion A for Alcohol Use Disorder.   The presence of at least two Criteria A1–A11 symptoms during the past 12 months is sufficient to meet criteria for Past-12-Month Alcohol Use Disorder. If this minimum threshold is met, severity specifiers (Mild, Moderate, and Severe) are also assigned based on the number of items that have been present during the past 12 months. The clinician then continues with the Past-12-Month Nonalcohol Substance Use Disorder section, starting with item label E14 on page 56.

10.7.2   Rating Past-12-Month Nonalcohol Substance Use Disorder (E14–E36)

This section begins with a determination of the patient's use of drugs or psychotropic medications in the past 12 months. The SCID-5-CV includes eight drug classes: Sedatives, Hypnotics, or Anxiolytics; Cannabis; Stimulants; Opioids; Phencyclidine and Related Substances; Other Hallucinogens; Inhalants; and Other (or Unknown). (Note that the listed order and configuration of the drug classes included in the SCID-5-CV differ from what is included in DSM-5. DSM-5 includes both Phencyclidine and Other Hallucinogens in a single drug class called "Hallucinogen-Related Disorders"; it also includes separate drug classes for tobacco and caffeine, which are not covered in the SCID. Moreover, DSM-5 lists the drug classes in alphabetical order, whereas the order of drug classes in the SCID was chosen to maintain continuity with earlier versions of the SCID.)

Starting with item label E15, the clinician asks the patient about his or her use of substances in each of the eight drug classes included in the SCID-5-CV. If the patient indicates having used a drug from that class in the past 12 months, the clinician should circle the "YES" rating for that drug class and write in the name of any specific drug used. If the patient credibly denies having used any drug in the past 12 months, then the clinician continues the SCID-5-CV with item label F1, the evaluation of Panic Disorder. For example, the first drug class inquired about are the sedatives, hypnotics, or anxiolytics: "In the past 12 months, have you taken any pills to calm you down, help you relax, or help you sleep? (Drugs like Valium, Xanax, Ativan, Klonopin, Ambien, Sonata, or Lunesta?)" If the patient responds by saying that he has regularly been taking Ambien for sleep during the past 12 months, the clinician would record "Ambien" in the indicated space and circle the "YES" rating in the right-hand column. If the patient acknowledges using any substance from any class (i.e., one of the ratings for item labels E15–E22 is "YES"), the clinician should continue the substance use assessment on the next page in order to determine whether the substance use exceeded the minimum threshold requirement needed to justify an assessment of the criteria for Substance Use Disorder for that class of substance.

For the next set of ratings (item labels E15a–E22a), the clinician determines for any drug class used in the past 12 months whether the drug use exceeded a minimum threshold, which indicates the need to assess for a Substance Use Disorder. If the amount of drug use is below that minimum threshold for all drug classes, then the clinician can skip out of the Substance Use Disorder assessment and continue with item label F1, the assessment of Panic Disorder.

The threshold set for illegal or recreational drugs is six times in the past 12 months. If that threshold is met for a drug class, the clinician then follows up with additional questions about the amount of drug use and the consequences of that use (e.g., "During the past year, when were you taking (SUBSTANCE) the most?" "How much were you using?" "Did your use of (SUBSTANCE) cause problems for you?"). The threshold used for prescribed or over-the-counter (OTC) medication is not based on the number of times the patient has taken medication, but on whether the patient was abusing it: "Over the past 12 months, did you get hooked or become dependent on (PRESCRIBED /OTC MEDICATION)? Did you ever take more of it than was prescribed or run out of your prescription early? Did you ever have to go to more than one doctor to make sure you didn't run out?"

Before evaluating Criteria A1–A11 for Nonalcohol Substance Use Disorder (beginning with item label E23), the clinician needs to determine which drug class to focus on first in those cases in which the patient has used multiple drugs in the past 12 months. Therefore in the box just above item label E23, the clinician asks the following questions: "Which drugs or medications caused you the most problems over the past 12 months, since (ONE YEAR AGO)? Which ones did you use the most? Which were your 'drugs of choice'?" Based on the patient's answers, the clinician should select the drug class that is most likely to result in a diagnosis of Substance Use Disorder. If it turns out that the criteria are not met for Substance Use Disorder for that drug class, the clinician will be asked to reassess Criteria A1–A11 for the other drug classes that are potentially likely to lead to a diagnosis of Substance Use Disorder.

Criterion A1—Larger amounts/longer periods than intended.   The intent of this item is to capture the patient's failed attempts to put some limits on his or her drug use (e.g., "I'm just going to have a couple of hits tonight"). Note that the breaking of these self-imposed limits (e.g., the patient ends up smoking a whole joint) must occur OFTEN in order to be coded "+". There is something of a paradox inherent in the evaluation of this item (and Criterion A2 as well). For this criterion to apply, the patient must have developed enough insight about having a drug use problem (or wanting to avoid developing a drug use problem) to want to control his or her drug use. Criterion A1 does not receive a "+" rating if someone has a very heavy pattern of use but denies any need to control or cut down use. For example, heavy users of cannabis may be unlikely to attempt to cut down or control their use of the substance because of their perception that cannabis is harmless.

Criterion A2—Persistent desire or failed efforts to cut down/control substance use.   This item is rated "+" under two circumstances. First, if the patient has had a persistent desire to stop, cut down, or control his or her drug use, presumably because of a self-awareness that it has been problematic in some way, a rating of "+" would apply. Although DSM-5 leaves the definition of "persistent" up to clinical judgment, a period lasting at least 1 month in which the person's desire to cut back or control substance use occurred for most of the time would be a reasonable minimum duration to count as "persistent." Second, in cases in which the patient does not have a persistent desire to cut down or control substance use but nonetheless has tried unsuccessfully to cut down or control drug use (e.g., in response to repeated demands from family members), a rating of "+" would also apply. Note that for an effort to cut down or control substance use to be considered "successful" (and justify a rating of "—"), the period of controlled or diminished use must have lasted for an extended period of time (e.g., months or years).

Criterion A3—Great deal of time spent on substance use.   This item covers the various ways in which drug use may become a central focus of the patient's life. This is especially variable across the classes of drugs because of differences in cost, availability, legality, and the typical pattern of use of a particular substance. For example, the high cost, daily need, and relative unavailability of opioids is much more likely to result in an individual becoming totally preoccupied with the daily task of procuring them. In contrast, this item is less likely to apply to inhalants because of their low cost, wide availability in stores, and the typical pattern of intermittent use.

Reasonable people may disagree about what constitutes "a great deal of time." As a rule of thumb, two evenings a week spent smoking pot is not "a great deal of time" and probably justifies a rating of "—"; being high every day certainly would justify a rating of "+".

Criterion A4—Craving.   Criterion A4 assesses the strong urge or desire to use the substance at times when the substance is not actually being used. The intensity threshold for craving should be such that the craving has some negative impact on the patient. For example, the urge to use the substance might be so strong that the patient has trouble thinking about anything else, or it results in significant discomfort or greatly weakens the patient's resolve to cut back on or quit using the substance. In some patients, the urge to use the substance is associated with specific cues, like seeing drug paraphernalia or running into a buddy on the street with whom the patient has used drugs. To explore this typical trigger for craving, the follow-up question asks whether the craving is associated with certain situations.

Criterion A5—Failure to fulfill obligations at work, school, or home.   A rating of "+" for this item requires specific evidence that the effects of the substance use (i.e., intoxication, withdrawal, hangover) resulted in the patient's failure to fulfill a major role obligation on at least two occasions. The accompanying examples illustrate the wide range of the types of activities that may be affected: repeated absences from work or poor work performance; absences, suspensions, or expulsions from school; and neglect of children or household responsibilities. Simply being high while at work, school, or taking care of children without apparent impairment is not sufficient to justify a rating of "+"; there must be some evidence that the effects of the substance significantly and recurrently interfered with functioning in one of these domains.

Criterion A6—Continued use despite recurrent interpersonal problems as a result of substance use. Like Criterion A5, Criterion A6 reflects social or interpersonal problems that are caused by the effects of substance use, such as marital strain caused by arguments or physical fights that occur during periods of intoxication. Unlike Criterion A5, a "+" rating for Criterion A6 requires that the patient continue to use the substance despite these problems. Criterion A6 may be difficult to evaluate when the interpersonal conflict is possibly attributable to an underlying relational problem rather than to a problem with the individual's substance use. For example, arguments about occasional nonproblematic substance use that are initiated by a spouse who believes that even minimal drug use is intolerable would not warrant a rating of "+".

Criterion A7—Important activities given up at work, school, or home so that time can be spent on substance use. The prototypical patient whose substance use meets this criterion is a heroin addict who has essentially given up all activities except those associated with procuring and using heroin. However, Criterion A7 may also apply, for example, to an amateur athlete who has stopped sports activities because of substance use or to a person who has stopped seeing all her friends so she can stay home and get "high."

Criterion A8—Recurrent use in physically hazardous situations. A common error in rating this item is to be overinclusive and assume that any level of substance use in a situation that requires alertness would qualify. The item should be rated "+" only if the substance use caused sufficient impairment in coordination or cognition to create a physically hazardous situation (e.g., driving or hunting while high on a substance). To facilitate a proper inquiry, the first question simply establishes that the patient has used the substance before engaging in an activity that requires coordination and concentration. If the patient acknowledges such use, the follow-up question then establishes whether the patient was in fact impaired to a degree that someone could have been injured as a result of the impaired coordination or concentration.

It is important to take into account the type of substance and the amount used to infer the likely level of impairment associated with its use, a judgment that works both ways. For example, the benefit of the doubt might be given to someone who says, for example, that he can drive perfectly well after using a "bump" of cocaine. On the other hand, if someone admits to taking a high dose of hallucinogens and insists that he or she was not impaired, the clinician may choose to rate a "+" nonetheless.

Although getting stoned and walking home through a dangerous neighborhood or having unprotected sex with someone one doesn't know very well while intoxicated is certainly risky, neither would warrant a rating of "+"; the intent of this item is to rate behavior that puts the patient or others in immediate danger because his or her coordination or cognition is impaired by the substance.

Criterion A9—Continued use despite knowledge that physical or psychological problems are caused or made worse by the substance. Like Criterion A6, Criterion A9 is meant to tap a pattern of compulsive use of the substance and does not refer merely to the adverse physical or psychological consequences of using the substance. Consequently, for the clinician to rate this item "+", the patient must first acknowledge understanding that the physical or psychological problems that he or she is experiencing are caused by use of the substance and that despite this knowledge, he or she has been unable to stop using it or cut down significantly. Examples of physical problems include serious damage to nasal mucosa from sniffing cocaine or exacerbation of asthma from smoking excessive amounts of marijuana. Examples of psychological problems are cocaine-induced paranoia or panic attacks precipitated by marijuana.

Criterion A10—Tolerance. Tolerance is the need for a person to use greater amounts of a substance to get the same effect as when that person first started using it. Although the criterion requires the need for "markedly increased amounts," how much the amount needs to have increased is left up to clinical judgment. The DSM-III-R version of the tolerance criterion specified at least a 50% increase, but this requirement was dropped from DSM-IV because it was felt to be pseudoprecise. Tolerance develops most frequently with amphetamines, cocaine, opioids, and sedatives (especially barbiturates). Tolerance for many drugs (e.g. cocaine, barbiturates, heroin) is usually apparent to the patient. It may not be possible to establish tolerance for drugs like marijuana, where the quality of the drug varies markedly.

Criterion A11—Withdrawal. Withdrawal is indicated by the development of the characteristic substance-specific withdrawal syndrome (in the List of Withdrawal Symptoms at the end of Module E) shortly after stopping or decreasing the amount of the substance. In some cases, the individual never allows the withdrawal syndrome to develop because he or she starts taking more of the substance in anticipation of the onset of withdrawal symptoms. The severity and clinical significance of the withdrawal syndrome varies by class of substance. Characteristic withdrawal syndromes are most apparent with sedatives and opioids. Based on DSM-5 criteria, symptoms of withdrawal syndromes are provided for the following drug classes: sedatives, hypnotics, or anxiolytics; cannabis; stimulants (including cocaine); and opioids. Because DSM-5 (Table 1, p. 482) does not recognize withdrawal from PCP, hallucinogens, or inhalants, the SCID-5-CV likewise omits these drug classes from withdrawal syndromes.

Meeting Criterion A for Nonalcohol Substance Use Disorder. The presence of at least two Criteria A1–A11 symptoms for the same substance during the past 12 months is sufficient to meet criteria for Past-12-Month Nonalcohol Substance Use Disorder. If the two-symptom minimum threshold is met for use of a specific substance, the clinician gives a "YES" rating for item label E35 and continues with item label E36 on page 61, where the specific type and severity of the Nonalcohol Substance Use Disorder is determined. The clinician indicates the diagnosis by circling the specific substance use disorder and its severity level; the clinician also records the name of the specific drug. (The diagnosis depends on the current severity, which can be Mild, Moderate, or Severe, depending on the number of items that have been present during the past 12 months. The corresponding diagnostic code for the type and severity of the substance use disorder is recorded on the Diagnostic Summary Score Sheet, along with the name of the specific drug.) If the minimum threshold of two items is not met for the drug class being assessed, the clinician gives a "NO" rating for item label E35 and follows the arrow down to the instruction that asks the clinician to consider whether there has been evidence of clinically significant use of another drug class (from item labels E15–E22) other than the one that was just assessed, for which criteria were not met. If so, the clinician will need to return to item label E23 at the top of page 58 and go through the Nonalcohol Substance Use Disorder items again, but this time focusing on the other drug class, given that the use pattern assessed for the first drug class was not severe enough to meet criteria. If and only if there are no other drug classes for which there is the possibility of a Past-12-Month Nonalcohol Substance Use Disorder should the clinician then skip out at this point and continue with the assessment of Panic Disorder, starting with item label F1 on page 63.

10.8   Module F.   Anxiety Disorders

10.8.1   Ratings for Panic Disorder (F1–F22)

Criteria for panic attack.   The term "panic attack" is often incorrectly used by patients to describe any escalating anxiety. A true *panic attack* is characterized by a sudden and intense rush of physical manifestations of anxiety combined with cognitions such as a fear of dying or losing control. Immediately after establishing the characteristic crescendo of anxiety and before going through the individual symptoms, the clinician asks the patient to provide a description of the last bad panic attack that he or she has experienced. This serves several functions. First, it provides an opportunity for the patient to describe the attack and its accompanying symptoms in his or her own words before being cued with the list of 13 panic attack symptoms. Second, it allows the clinician to more easily determine whether the course of the reported anxiety episode is consistent with a true panic attack (i.e., an abrupt surge of intense fear that reaches a peak within minutes), rather than a more extended period of anxiety that might be more consistent with Generalized Anxiety Disorder. Finally, the determination of whether at least four symptoms occurred together during the same panic attack is facilitated by asking the patient to think about a specific attack when answering the questions about the individual symptoms. One potential pitfall of this approach is that if the threshold of four symptoms is not reached, it may be because the panic attack chosen by the patient may not be the most severe one that the person has experienced. Thus, in cases in which the four-symptom threshold is not reached, the clinician needs to ask if there have been any more severe panic attacks in terms of the number of symptoms. If so, the clinician will need to apply the list of symptoms to this more severe panic attack and then, if the four-symptom threshold is met, confirm that such attacks have occurred at least twice. If the patient has not had four panic attack symptoms occurring together at any other time, the clinician is instructed to skip to the assessment of Agoraphobia in item label F23.

Criterion A—Recurrent unexpected panic attacks.

The presence of a panic attack is not necessarily indicative of Panic Disorder because panic attacks can occur in the context of a number of other disorders. For example, if a person with a snake phobia goes on a hike and has a panic attack after encountering a snake, this would not warrant an additional diagnosis of Panic Disorder. By definition, at least two of the panic attacks in Panic Disorder must have been "unexpected." Thus, the initial question explicitly asks whether the panic attack came on "out of the blue" (i.e., in a situation in which the patient would not have expected to be nervous or anxious, such as sitting at home watching TV). If the patient answers "YES," this is confirmed by asking the patient to describe the context in which the attack occurred. However, it is not uncommon for individuals with Panic Disorder to fairly quickly (and mistakenly) assume that there is a cause-and-effect relationship between the situations in which the attacks have developed and the attacks themselves and thus deny that any of the attacks have come on out of the blue. Therefore, there are explicit follow-up questions asking about the context of the initial panic attacks in order to determine if at least two of them were unexpected.

For some individuals, attacks may occur following a frightening thought, such as worrying that something terrible will happen to them or to a loved one. Such attacks should still be regarded as "unexpected" because the concept of "unexpected" refers to the absence of a clear association between an environmental stimulus and the occurrence of a panic attack. Common sense (we hope) will lead the clinician not to include as "unexpected" panic attacks that occur in response to unexpected but realistic dangers, such as being mugged. Similarly, panic attacks that occur in response to delusions about being harmed should not be regarded as "unexpected."

Criterion B—Worry about having another attack and/or maladaptive change in behavior.

This criterion ensures that the panic attacks have a negative impact on the person's life, which can be manifested in either of two ways. The patient may experience persistent concern or worry (lasting at least 1 month) about having additional attacks or about "their consequences," which has been interpreted in the SCID-5-CV to mean that the patient is worried about those symptoms that represent consequences of the attack, such as having a heart attack, losing control, or "going crazy." Alternatively, the patient may start avoiding places or situations that he or she believes might trigger a panic attack or else might make escape difficult in the event of having a panic attack. This avoidance may range from simply not driving a car because the person is afraid of having an attack while driving, all the way to never leaving home because of fear of having an attack in a place that's not "safe," possibly justifying an additional diagnosis of Agoraphobia.

Criterion C—Not due to a GMC and not substance/medication-induced.   This item instructs the clinician to consider and rule out a GMC or a substance/medication as an etiological cause of the panic attacks, in which case Anxiety Disorder Due to Another Medical Condition or Substance/Medication-Induced Anxiety Disorder is diagnosed. Remember to carefully assess caffeine intake, and remember that caffeine is present in a variety of foods, beverages, and over-the-counter medications such as headache remedies. (Caffeine is listed as one of the diagnostic codes for Substance-Induced Anxiety Disorder.) Although substance use may be associated with the initial onset of panic attacks, a substance-induced etiology should be considered when subsequent panic attacks occur ONLY in the context of substance use. See Section 9, "Differentiating General Medical and Substance/Medication Etiologies From Primary Disorders," in this User's Guide for a discussion of how to rate this criterion. If the clinician decides that the diagnosis is Anxiety Disorder Due to Another Medical Condition or Substance/Medication-Induced Anxiety Disorder, that diagnosis should be recorded in the Diagnostic Summary Score Sheet Score Sheet under Other Disorders.

Criterion D—Not better explained by another mental disorder.   This criterion covers essentially the same diagnostic ground as the requirement that there be at least two panic attacks that are unexpected. It asks whether the panic attacks are better accounted for by another mental disorder. This judgment depends on determining whether the panic attacks are cued by an anxiety-provoking stimulus arising in the context of another disorder. For example, consider an individual with long-standing Social Anxiety Disorder who has a panic attack while speaking in front of a large group of people. Because the panic attack was triggered by exposure to an anxiety-provoking situation (i.e., speaking in public), it is considered to be better explained by the diagnosis of Social Anxiety Disorder.

Rating for current Panic Disorder.   The assessment of the Panic Disorder criteria up to this point has focused on lifetime Panic Disorder. This item serves to determine whether criteria are currently met for Panic Disorder (i.e., in the past month). Rather than repeating the assessment of each Panic Disorder criterion for the current month, the SCID-5-CV only requires a determination of whether or not there have been at least two panic attacks in the past month or whether during the past month there has been either worry about having another panic attack (Criterion B1) or maladaptive changes in behavior related to the attacks (Criterion B2). Note that when assessing the presence of current panic attacks, it is not required that the panic attacks that have occurred in the past month be "unexpected," as the DSM-5 diagnosis of Panic Disorder requires only that at least two panic attacks during the individual's lifetime were unexpected. For the purposes of determining whether the Panic Disorder is current, recurrent panic attacks cued by places or situations would count, reflecting the typical course of Panic Disorder in which panic attacks subsequent to the initial unexpected panic attacks become associated with environmental triggers.

10.8.2   Ratings for Agoraphobia (F23–F31)

Agoraphobia is an Anxiety Disorder characterized by fear and avoidance of multiple types of places or situations because of a fear of having panic-like symptoms and thoughts that escape would be difficult or help not available. In contrast to DSM-IV, in which Agoraphobia was explicitly linked to Panic Disorder, in DSM-5 Agoraphobia is diagnosed separately from Panic Disorder, so both diagnoses are possible.

Criterion A—Fear or avoidance about at least two out of five types of situations. The first criterion for Agoraphobia in DSM-5 requires fear or anxiety about two (or more) out of five specific listed situations. In item label F23, the initial question to be asked is whether the patient has ever been "very anxious about or afraid of situations like going out of the house alone, being in crowds, going to stores, standing in lines, or traveling on buses or trains," which is followed by an open-ended inquiry into the actual types of situations that the patient has feared. This is followed by five specific questions asking about the five types of situations specified in the criterion (i.e., using public transportation, being in open spaces, being in enclosed spaces, standing in line or being in a crowd, being outside of the home alone). Note that these questions are preceded by the conditional instruction "IF UNKNOWN" because it is expected that most of the time after the initial question and the open-ended follow-up question the answers to these specific questions will already be known.

Criterion B—Fear or avoidance of situations due to thoughts that escape might be difficult or help might not be available.   The assessment of this criterion involves determining the reason that the patient is avoiding the situations in Criterion A. The first question is open-ended and asks why the patient is avoiding the situations and/ or what it is that the patient is afraid would happen if he or she were in one of those situations. Follow-up questions specifically cover the most common experiences, including being afraid that it would be hard to get out of the situation in case of having a panic attack, developing a symptom that would be embarrassing, becoming impaired in some way, or being worried that there would be nobody there to help if one of these incapacitating or embarrassing symptoms suddenly developed.

Criterion C—The agoraphobic situations almost always provoke fear or anxiety. This criterion reflects the phobic nature of the disturbance, requiring relative consistency with regard to the patient's reaction when in a feared situation. Thus, an individual who becomes anxious only occasionally in an agoraphobic situation (e.g., becomes anxious when standing in line on only one out of every five occasions) would not be diagnosed as having Agoraphobia. However, the degree of fear or anxiety expressed may vary, from anticipatory anxiety to a full panic attack, across different occasions of being in or anticipating being in a feared situation because of various contextual factors, such as the presence of a trusted companion.

Criterion D—The agoraphobic situations are actively avoided, require the presence of a companion, or are endured with intense fear or anxiety.   Note that a rating of "+" can still be appropriate for a patient who is able to force himself or herself to go into the feared situations, but only with either marked distress or an accompanying companion.

Criterion E—The fear or anxiety is out of proportion to the actual threat posed by the social situations and the sociocultural context.   This criterion requires the clinician to consider contextual or cultural factors that might indicate that the fear, anxiety, or avoidance is normal given the context. For example, it would not be appropriate to diagnose Agoraphobia in an individual who avoids going outside at night as a reasonable response to living in an extremely dangerous neighborhood. The SCID-5-CV addresses this component of the criterion directly by having the clinician ask the patient whether he or she feels any danger or threat to his or her safety when in the feared situations. Avoidance behavior based on cultural factors (e.g., prohibitions against women traveling alone in certain Muslim countries) also would not count toward the diagnosis, but there is no all-purpose question to cover all such scenarios—the clinician should apply this component of the criterion as appropriate, based on the cultural context of the patient.

Criterion F—The fear, anxiety, or avoidance is persistent.   A minimum duration of 6 months is required to rule out transient responses.

Criterion G—The fear, anxiety, or avoidance causes clinically significant distress or impairment.   Throughout the SCID-5-CV, "clinically significant distress or impairment" is assessed by asking an open-ended question to determine the impact that the fear, anxiety, or avoidance behavior has had on the patient's life. The follow-up questions are optional and specifically cover various domains of functioning that might be impacted by the fear, anxiety, or avoidance; they should be asked only if it is not clear from the patient's answer whether the symptoms interfere with functioning.

Criterion H—If a GMC is present, related fear, anxiety, or avoidance is excessive.   A number of GMCs, such as inflammatory bowel disease, Parkinson's disease, and severe coronary artery disease, are characterized by symptoms that at times can be physically incapacitating. Individuals with such medical conditions may appropriately avoid places or situations in which help might not be available in case of developing an incapacitating symptom related to one of these medical conditions, and in such cases a diagnosis of Agoraphobia should not be made. However, if the patient's fear, anxiety, or avoidance is clearly excessive, then the diagnosis is allowed. For example, avoiding driving for several weeks following a severe heart attack would certainly not warrant a diagnosis of Agoraphobia, whereas being housebound for 2 years following a mild heart attack might warrant the diagnosis.

Criterion I—Not better explained by another mental disorder.   This criterion is similar to Criterion D in Panic Disorder and serves as a reminder to consider whether the fear and avoidance may be better characterized as part of another mental disorder. Two of the most difficult boundaries for Agoraphobia are between Specific Phobia and Social Anxiety Disorder. Agoraphobia involves avoidance of at least two different types of situations, reflecting the general unpredictability of panic attacks. In contrast, Specific Phobia tends to be limited to one consistently feared situation. Furthermore, the onset of Agoraphobia is usually related to the onset of panic attacks, whereas Specific Phobia tends to be either lifelong or develops after a traumatic experience. Determining whether avoidance of social situations is related to Social Anxiety Disorder or to fear of developing a panic attack in a social situation (which could warrant a diagnosis of Agoraphobia) generally depends on the temporal relationship between the onset of panic attacks and the social avoidance. If an individual develops avoidance of social situations only AFTER the onset of panic attacks, then Agoraphobia is the most appropriate diagnosis. An individual with long-standing social avoidance who newly develops panic attacks when in social situations would better be considered to have Social Anxiety Disorder. Note that this criterion does NOT preclude making a diagnosis of BOTH Agoraphobia and another disorder characterized by avoidance in the same individual (e.g., an individual with a long-standing dog phobia since childhood who develops unexpected panic attacks in situations without the presence of dogs).

10.8.3   Ratings for Social Anxiety Disorder (Social Phobia) (F32–F41)

Criterion A—Marked fear or anxiety about one or more social situations.   A wide range of social triggers may qualify for the "social situations" in this criterion—what they all have in common is that the person is exposed to the scrutiny of others. Three types of situations are included: social interactions, such as having a conversation or meeting unfamiliar people; being observed by others eating, drinking, or going to the bathroom; or performing in front of others, such as giving a speech or a musical performance. Note that in order to rate this criterion "+", the degree of fear or anxiety must be "marked" (according to the DSM-5 criterion) or "intense" (according to the DSM-5 text, p. 203). Because concerns about public speaking are so ubiquitous, it is important to avoid rating this criterion as "+" for public speaking unless it is clear that the person's concerns are excessive and do not diminish with practice.

Criterion B—Fear of acting in a way that will be negatively evaluated.   This item establishes the reason for the fear of social situations. After starting out with an open-ended question (i.e., "What were you afraid would happen when…"), several follow-up questions covering specific reasons for the fear are offered if the patient's response to the initial question is unclear (e.g., "afraid of being embarrassed," "afraid [of…] being rejected," "making others uncomfortable or offending them"). This last example applies especially to individuals from cultures with strong collectivistic orientations (e.g., Japan). Avoidance of a behavior because of concerns that the person's own high standards will not be met (as in Obsessive-Compulsive Personality Disorder) would not warrant a rating of "+".

Criterion C—The social situations almost always provoke fear or anxiety.   This criterion should be rated "—" if the anxiety and avoidance are erratically expressed (e.g., fear of speaking in one class, but no fear of speaking in a different class with the same number of people).

Criterion D—Social situations are avoided or endured with intense fear or anxiety. This criterion demonstrates that avoidance of social situations is not a required part of this disorder. A diagnosis of Social Anxiety Disorder may also apply to those who force themselves to go to parties, give talks, or go on job interviews, but feel intensely anxious while doing it.

Criterion E—The fear or anxiety is out of proportion to the actual threat posed by the social situations and to the sociocultural context. This criterion requires the clinician to consider contextual or cultural factors that might indicate that the patient's social anxiety is normal given the context. For example, it would not be appropriate to diagnose Social Anxiety Disorder in an individual whose avoidance of social situations is limited to those in which he or she is being bullied or threatened. Similarly, the diagnosis would not apply if an individual's performance anxiety were limited to situations in which a poor performance has serious negative consequences (e.g., high levels of fear and anxiety in anticipation of defending a thesis). Accordingly, the SCID-5-CV includes an open-ended question for asking the patient about his or her opinion of the likely impact of performing badly in the feared situation. The patient's answer would then be assessed to evaluate possible distortions about the likelihood of performing badly (e.g., the patient ignores the fact that he or she has extensively rehearsed) or possible exaggeration about the impact of failing. Avoidance behavior based on cultural factors (e.g., cultural expectations that women be reticent in social situations) also would not count toward the diagnosis, but there is no all-purpose question to cover all such scenarios—the clinician should apply this component of the criterion as appropriate, based on the cultural context of the patient.

Criterion F—The fear, anxiety, or avoidance is persistent. A minimum duration of 6 months is required to rule out transient responses.

Criterion G—The fear, anxiety, or avoidance causes clinically significant distress or impairment. Throughout the SCID-5-CV, "clinically significant distress or impairment" is assessed by asking an open-ended question to determine the impact that the fear, anxiety, or avoidance behavior has had on the patient's life. The follow-up questions are optional and specifically cover various domains of functioning that might be impacted by the fear, anxiety, or avoidance; they should be asked only if it is not clear from the patient's answer whether the symptoms interfere with functioning.

Most potential diagnoses of Social Anxiety Disorder sink or swim on this "clinical significance" criterion. Master SCIDers may choose to skip directly to the rating of this criterion if it seems likely that the social anxiety is going to turn out to be clinically insignificant. A diagnosis of Social Anxiety Disorder is not made unless the avoidance, anticipatory anxiety, or distress is clinically significant (i.e., interferes with functioning, with social activities, or with relationships; or there is marked distress ABOUT having the fear or avoidance). Thus, for example, a fear of public speaking in a plumber who is almost never called upon to address groups of people is unlikely to meet this criterion. Some individuals who seriously constrict their lives to avoid social situations may report a lack of distress because their social anxiety is so rarely activated. A rating of "+" may still be justified if the clinician makes a judgment that the social anxiety has had a significant negative impact on such patients' functioning.

Criterion H—Not due to a GMC and not substance/medication-induced. The type of anxiety or avoidance seen in Social Anxiety Disorder would rarely be associated with a GMC or substance/medication. It is possible, however, to imagine a scenario in which the patient who uses excessive amounts of caffeine or amphetamine to enhance his or her cognitive performance in social situations has anxiety in such situations that is due to the substance use rather than the social situation itself. See Section 9, "Differentiating General Medical and Substance/Medication Etiologies From Primary Disorders," in this User's Guide for a discussion of how to rate this criterion. If the clinician decides that the diagnosis is Anxiety Disorder Due to Another Medical Condition or Substance/Medication-Induced Anxiety Disorder, that diagnosis should be recorded in the Diagnostic Summary Score Sheet under Other Disorders.

Criterion I—Not better explained by another mental disorder. This criterion is similar to Criterion I in Agoraphobia, in that it serves as a reminder to consider whether the fear and avoidance may be better characterized as part of another mental disorder. Although not explicitly mentioned in Criterion I, one of the more difficult boundaries to determine is between Social Anxiety Disorder and Agoraphobia. Typically, Agoraphobia involves avoidance of a cluster of situations, reflecting the general unpredictability of panic attacks. Determining whether avoidance of social situations is related to Social Anxiety Disorder or to fear of developing a panic attack in a social situation (which would warrant a diagnosis of Agoraphobia) generally depends on determining the temporal relationship between the onset of panic attacks and the social avoidance. If an individual develops social avoidance only AFTER the onset of panic attacks, then Agoraphobia is the most appropriate diagnosis. A patient with long-standing social avoidance who develops panic attacks when in social situations would better be considered to have Social Anxiety Disorder. Although also not explicitly mentioned in Criterion I, other anxiety disorders are differentiated from Social Anxiety Disorder by virtue of the focus of the anxiety (e.g., in Separation Anxiety Disorder, the anxiety is related to being separated from attachment figures, rather than being triggered by social situations).

Criterion J—If a GMC or potentially embarrassing mental disorder is present, the fear, anxiety, or avoidance is clearly unrelated or is excessive. A number of GMCs (e.g., Parkinson's disease, obesity, disfigurement from burns or injuries) and mental disorders (e.g., Tic Disorder, Childhood-Onset Fluency Disorder [Stuttering], Anorexia Nervosa) are characterized by symptoms that are embarrassing and could potentially lead to social ostracism. Thus, it may be reasonable for some individuals with such medical conditions or mental disorders to avoid social situations because of the real possibility that they will be embarrassed or rejected; such individuals should not be diagnosed with Social Anxiety Disorder. However, the clinician can still make a diagnosis of Social Anxiety Disorder if, according to his or her judgment, the patient's fear or anxiety about the social situation either 1) is clearly unrelated to the patient's medical condition or mental disorder or 2) is excessive. Note that the bracketed phrase "or potentially embarrassing mental disorder" is not in the DSM-5 criterion and has been added to the SCID-5-CV. The corresponding DSM-IV Criterion H ("If a general medical condition or other mental disorder is present, the fear…is unrelated to it, e.g., the fear is not of Stuttering, trembling in Parkinson's disease, or exhibiting abnormal eating behavior in Anorexia Nervosa or Bulimia Nervosa") included both GMCs and mental disorders. After discussion with the DSM-5 Work Group, it was determined that the mental disorder component was unintentionally omitted from this criterion.

10.8.4   Ratings for Current Generalized Anxiety Disorder (F42–F54)

Criterion A—Excessive anxiety and worry about a variety of events and activities, more days than not.   Separate questions are provided for each of the three subcomponents of this criterion that all must be true in order for the criterion to be rated "+". First, the anxiety and worry are not focused on one or two issues, but instead involve a wide range of issues. For example, such an individual worries about the health and safety of his spouse and children, his financial situation, the possibility of being late for an appointment, not having enough time to finish a project, what to wear to a party, whether his job is in jeopardy, and whether there are jellyfish in the water. Second, the anxiety and worry must be "excessive"—that is, the intensity, duration, or frequency of the anxiety and worry is out of proportion to the actual likelihood or impact of the anticipated event (e.g., an individual is preoccupied with worries about a 30-year-old spouse dying from a heart attack, despite absence of medical problems aside from mild cholesterol elevation). Finally, the anxiety and worry must have occurred for more days than not during the past 6 months.

Criterion B—Worry is difficult to control.   Recognizing that the worry is excessive, individuals with this problem will often tell themselves to stop it and will try to think about something else, but will find themselves drifting inexorably back to whatever worry is preoccupying them at the time.

Criterion C—Three of six associated symptoms.   Note that like the generalized anxiety itself, some of these symptoms must also be present "more days than not" for a period of at least 6 months.

Criterion D—Causes clinically significant distress or impairment.   This criterion helps to set the boundary between the clinically significant anxiety in Generalized Anxiety Disorder and "normal" anxiety. The anxiety and worry should be considered clinically significant only if they are sufficiently severe to cause marked distress or impairment in functioning.

Criterion E—Not due to a GMC and not substance/medication-induced. GMCs and substances/medications must be considered and ruled out as etiological factors for the anxiety, in which case Anxiety Disorder Due to Another Medical Condition or Substance/Medication-Induced Anxiety Disorder is diagnosed. Remember to carefully assess caffeine intake, bearing in mind that caffeine is present in a variety of foods, beverages, and over-the-counter medications such as headache remedies. See Section 9, "Differentiating General Medical and Substance/Medication Etiologies From Primary Disorders," in this User's Guide for a discussion of how to rate this criterion. If the clinician decides that the diagnosis is Anxiety Disorder Due to Another Medical Condition or Substance/Medication-Induced Anxiety Disorder, that diagnosis should be recorded in the Diagnostic Summary Score Sheet under Other Disorders.

Criterion F—Not better explained by another mental disorder. Anxiety and worry are important components of many mental disorders. A diagnosis of Generalized Anxiety Disorder is appropriate only if there are additional symptoms of anxiety and foci of worry that are not part of another mental disorder. For example, an individual with prominent social anxiety who is preoccupied by worry about being embarrassed in social situations might warrant an additional diagnosis of Generalized Anxiety Disorder if there are also worries about health, financial, and other nonsocial issues.

10.9   Module G.   Obsessive-Compulsive Disorder and Posttraumatic Stress Disorder

In the SCID-5-RV, OCD is included in its own module along with the other DSM-5 Obsessive-Compulsive and Related Disorders, reflecting their grouping in DSM-5. Similarly, in the SCID-5-RV, PTSD is included in its own module along with the other DSM-5 Trauma- and Stressor-Related Disorders, such as Acute Stress Disorder. Given that these other disorders are not covered in the SCID-5-CV, both OCD and PTSD are presented together in Module G. (Grouped in DSM-5 with Trauma- and Stressor-Related Disorders, Adjustment Disorder is placed in its own module [Module J] at the very end of the SCID-5-CV. The evaluation of Adjustment Disorder in the SCID-5-CV follows that of all other disorders, because its diagnosis applies only if there is an identified stressor and criteria are not met for any other specific DSM-5 disorder.)

10.9.1   Ratings for Obsessive-Compulsive Disorder (G1–G8)

Criterion A. *Obsessions (1)—recurrent and persistent thoughts, urges, or images.* *Obsessions* are defined as thoughts, urges, or images that are experienced at some time during the disturbance as intrusive and unwanted. A patient's experience of these thoughts, urges, or images may change over the course of the disturbance; hence, the DSM inclusion of the phrase "at some time during the disturbance." The SCID-5-CV assessment of OCD begins with three questions to assess the different types of obsessions, along with a request for specifics if the patient answers "YES" to any of these:

- The first question queries for obsessions that take the form of <u>thoughts</u>: "Have you been bothered by thoughts that kept coming back to you even when you didn't want them to, like being exposed to germs or dirt or needing everything to be lined up in a certain way?"
- The second question queries for <u>obsessive images</u>: "How about having images popping into your head that you didn't want, like violent or horrible scenes or something of a sexual nature?"
- The third question queries for <u>obsessive urges</u>: "How about having urges to do something that kept coming back to you even though you didn't want them to, like an urge to harm a loved one?"

The most common diagnostic problem is distinguishing true obsessions from other repetitive distressing thoughts, such as excessive worries about realistic concerns, depressive ruminations, and delusions. Obsessions have an intrusive, inappropriate, and "ego-alien" quality and are experienced by the patient as something different and stranger than the worries or preoccupations that characterize Generalized Anxiety Disorder. A patient's recurrent, intrusive, and anxiety-provoking thought while driving that he or she ran over a small child without realizing it is an obsession. A patient spending an equal amount of time worrying about his or her retirement is more likely to be an aspect of Generalized Anxiety Disorder. Unlike obsessions, depressive ruminations and delusions are generally not perceived as intrusive or inappropriate, but are understood by the patient as a valid focus of concern, even if he or she realizes that the concern is excessive and tries to stop thinking about it.

In those situations in which the differential diagnosis is particularly challenging, it may be useful to remember the fact that obsessions and compulsions usually go together (in fact, more than 90% of the time according to the DSM-IV OCD field trial). Therefore, in trying to distinguish between an OCD obsession and other repetitive thoughts, the clinching point may be whether or not compulsions are also present.

After the three questions about types of obsessions, the follow-up question in item label G1 ("IF YES TO ANY OF ABOVE") asks whether the thoughts, urges, or images made the person upset. This aspect of the criterion (causing marked anxiety or distress) is not actually a requirement, given that the criterion specifies that the anxiety or distress is present for "most individuals." If the thoughts, urges, or images do <u>not</u> cause anxiety or distress, this does not rule out the diagnosis of an obsession; however, the presence of anxiety or distress will strengthen confidence in the existence of an obsession rather than another kind of repetitive thought.

Obsessions (2)—attempts to ignore, suppress, or neutralize. Another distinguishing feature of an obsession is that the individual tries to reduce the anxiety or distress associated with the thought, urge, or image by actively trying to ignore or suppress the thought (e.g., an individual with a contamination obsession avoiding known triggers such as dirt) or by neutralizing it by performing a compulsion.

Compulsions (1) and (2)—repetitive behaviors or mental acts. *Compulsions* are distinguished from other forms of repetitive behavior by the underlying motivation for the behavior: to reduce or prevent the anxiety associated with an obsession (e.g., hand washing alleviates the anxiety triggered by an obsession of being contaminated; repeating a prayer exactly 36 times is meant to counteract the distress caused by having an obsessive obscene thought). The patient's specific repetitive behaviors are queried in item label G3. The most common compulsions are behaviors like hand washing, repetitive touching or picking up and replacing an object repeatedly, or mental acts such as counting or repeating a word or phrase over and over.

Determining that the behavior is intended to reduce anxiety accompanying an obsession is very helpful in differentiating a compulsion from other repetitive behaviors such as tics and stereotypies. The first question in item label G4 addresses the purpose of the compulsions. The next questions in item label G4 ("How many times would you do (COMPULSIVE ACT)? Are you doing (COMPULSIVE ACT) more than really makes sense?") are intended to help the clinician determine whether the "behaviors or mental acts either are not connected in a realistic way with what they are designed to neutralize or prevent, or are clearly excessive," which is a required feature in addition to the requirement that the behaviors or mental acts are aimed at preventing or reducing distress. Even though the patient is asked whether he or she thinks the behavior "really makes sense," the judgment about whether the behaviors or acts are connected in a realistic way or are excessive is ultimately up to the clinician.

Check for obsessions and/or compulsions. The clinician moves on to the evaluation of Criterion B only if Criterion A is present. Thus, if there have never been any obsessions or compulsions, the clinician skips out of the assessment of OCD and moves on to the assessment of PTSD, starting with item G9, page 76.

Criterion B—Clinical significance.

This criterion requires that the obsessions or compulsions be clinically significant. Note that the clinical significance criterion also includes a phrase indicating that the obsessions or compulsions may be "time-consuming (e.g., take more than 1 hour per day)." This clause allows the clinician to conclude that impairment is present even in the face of the patient's apparent lack of concern or denial about the behavior or the rationalization that it is useful.

Criterion C—Not due to a GMC and not substance/medication-induced.

This item instructs the clinician to consider and rule out a GMC or a substance/medication as an etiological factor for the obsessions or compulsions. (Such etiologies are quite rare.) If either a GMC or a substance/medication is an etiological factor for the symptoms, Obsessive-Compulsive and Related Disorder Due to Another Medical Condition or Substance/Medication-Induced Obsessive-Compulsive and Related Disorder is diagnosed. See Section 9, "Differentiating General Medical and Substance/Medication Etiologies From Primary Disorders," in this User's Guide for a discussion of how to rate this criterion. If the clinician decides that the diagnosis is Obsessive-Compulsive and Related Disorder Due to Another Medical Condition or Substance/Medication-Induced Obsessive-Compulsive and Related Disorder, that diagnosis should be recorded in the Diagnostic Summary Score Sheet under Other Disorders.

Criterion D—Not better explained by another mental disorder. An additional diagnosis of OCD should not be given along with another mental disorder if the repetitive thoughts or behaviors can be considered features of the other mental disorder. Many of the symptoms of other disorders that are given as examples in the DSM-5 criterion do not really meet the OCD Criterion A test for obsessions as "intrusive and unwanted." For example, when a patient with Anorexia Nervosa is preoccupied with measuring the exact number of calories in the food she eats, she may agree only that it is excessive, but not that it is intrusive or unwanted. Of course, having Anorexia Nervosa does not protect someone against OCD; the patient with Anorexia Nervosa may also have hand-washing rituals that are unrelated to her eating disorder, and therefore be given both diagnoses.

10.9.2   Ratings for Posttraumatic Stress Disorder (G9–G41)

Lifetime Trauma History. Given that current PTSD can result from trauma exposure at any time during the patient's lifetime, the assessment of PTSD begins with a lifetime trauma history (item label G9) that corresponds to Criterion A in DSM-5. Five screening questions are provided that cover major types of trauma: 1) disasters, fires, combat, car accidents, and workplace accidents; 2) actual or threatened physical or sexual assault or abuse; 3) seeing another person being physically or sexually assaulted or abused, or threatened with physical or sexual assault; 4) seeing another person killed or dead, or badly hurt; and 5) learning that one of these things happened to someone the patient is close to. In order to capture instances of trauma exposure that might have been missed by these screening questions, an additional question asks whether the patient has ever been a victim of a serious crime. Finally, if the patient has not endorsed any traumatic events thus far, the clinician concludes the trauma screening in item label G9 by asking the patient to describe the most stressful or traumatic experience ever in his or her life.

If there have been any traumatic events in the patient's lifetime, the clinician is instructed to inquire about three of the events using the detailed questions in the boxes for item labels G10–G12 (pages 76–77). For each event, the clinician first records the description of the event and then classifies the event in terms of the type of event (actual or threatened death, actual or threatened serious injury, actual or threatened sexual violence) and the mode of exposure (direct experience, witnessing in person it happening to others, learning about it happening to a close family member or friend, or repeated or extreme exposure to aversive details of traumatic events). Finally, for each event, the clinician indicates the patient's age at the time of the event and whether it was a single event or else prolonged or repeated exposure to the same trauma, such as ongoing domestic violence. The choice of the three events detailed in item labels G10–G12 is up to the clinician and could be the three "worst" events (i.e., most severe), the three most recent events, or any combination.

Note that in the process of deciding whether a traumatic experience qualifies for Criterion A (to be rated in item label G13), it is helpful to be aware of the scope of trauma examples that are included in the DSM-5 text:

> The directly experienced [qualifying] traumatic events in Criterion A include, but are not limited to, exposure to war as a combatant or civilian, threatened or actual physical assault (e.g., physical attack, robbery, mugging, childhood physical abuse), threatened or actual sexual violence (e.g., forced sexual penetration, alcohol/drug-facilitated sexual penetration, abusive sexual contact, noncontact sexual abuse, sexual trafficking), being kidnapped, being taken hostage, terrorist attack, torture, incarceration as a prisoner of war, natural or human-made disasters, and severe motor vehicle accidents. For children, sexually violent events may include developmentally inappropriate sexual experiences without physical violence or injury. (p. 274)

Regarding potentially traumatic medical incidents, DSM-5 points out that experiencing a life-threatening or debilitating medical problem does not necessarily qualify. According to DSM-5 (p. 274), "Medical incidents that qualify as traumatic events involve sudden, catastrophic events (e.g., waking during surgery, anaphylactic shock)."

With respect to the types of witnessed events that might qualify for Criterion A, according to DSM-5, such events

> include, but are not limited to, observing threatened or serious injury, unnatural death, physical or sexual abuse of another person due to violent assault, domestic violence, accident, war or disaster, or a medical catastrophe in one's child (e.g., a life-threatening hemorrhage). (p. 274)

Note that witnessing a natural death, such as being present in a hospital room during the death of a close friend or relative, is not a qualifying trauma. With respect to indirect exposure through learning about an event, according to DSM-5, qualifying traumas are

> limited to experiences affecting close relatives or friends and experiences that are violent or accidental (e.g., death due to natural causes does not qualify). Such events include violent personal assault, suicide, serious accident, and serious injury. (pp. 274–275)

Some of these traumatic events may be difficult for the patient to discuss, much less remember the details. If the clinician notices the patient hesitating or showing other signs of distress, it is important to attend to this difficulty. Often, a patient's discomfort is soothed by hearing why it is important to have details about the traumatic event(s) (e.g., "I know it might be hard for you to describe what happened. It's important for us to get as much detail as we can so that we can link your symptoms to a specific event that happened in your life, so I appreciate you providing the best information you can").

Criterion A—Exposure to actual or threatened death, serious injury, or sexual violence.   If the only traumatic events that the patient has been exposed to have occurred within the past month, the clinician is instructed to skip to the assessment of ADHD as criteria cannot be met for PTSD because of the greater than 1-month minimum duration of symptoms. (Such cases might meet criteria for Acute Stress Disorder, a diagnosis not covered in the SCID-5-CV). If the patient has been exposed to one or more traumatic events prior to the past month, the clinician is instructed to review the description of the traumatic events in item labels G10–G12 (pages 76–77) to verify that at least one of these traumatic events meets the requirement of Criterion A. If the patient has been exposed to more than one qualifying Criterion A event, the clinician should determine which event has had the greatest impact on the patient by asking, "Which of these…do you think has affected you the most?"

The patient is asked which event (from item labels G10–G12) had the greatest impact on him or her so that the clinician can select the event for the assessment of symptomatic response that is most likely to meet the criteria for PTSD. However, after proceeding through the PTSD criteria (item labels G13–G41), it is certainly possible that one of the other events could also have resulted in PTSD. Therefore, if the response to the selected event does not end up meeting full criteria for PTSD and there were other reported traumas in item labels G10–G12, the clinician should cycle through the PTSD criteria set again, using one of these other traumatic events for the purpose of assessing the PTSD criteria.

After Criterion A, remaining items in the PTSD criteria set are each first rated for whether the symptom has occurred during the period of time dating from the exposure to the traumatic event up to the present (lifetime PTSD). Then for each item rated "+", the clinician follows up with a question (e.g., "Has this also been the case in the past month?") in order to determine whether the symptom was present during the past month (current PTSD). The past-month ratings for each item are necessary in order to determine whether the full criteria for PTSD have been met currently (i.e., in the past month).

Criterion B—At least one intrusion symptom.   It is important to make sure that the symptoms developed for the first time after exposure to the traumatic event.

Criterion B1—Involuntary and intrusive distressing memories of event.   This item requires that the patient has experienced involuntary and intrusive memories of the event. The memories usually include sensory, emotional, or physiological behavioral components. Intrusive recollections are distinguished from depressive ruminations (which, given the high rates of comorbidity with depression, may also be present) in that they are experienced by the person as involuntary and unwelcome.

Criterion B2—Dreams of the event.   The distressing dreams that would qualify for a rating of "+" are not necessarily limited to those that replay the event itself but also include dream content or affect that is representative or thematically related to the major threats involved in the traumatic event.

Criterion B3—Dissociative reactions in which event is reexperienced. The person experiences dissociative states that can last from a few seconds to several hours or even days, during which aspects of the event are relived and the person feels or acts as if the event were occurring at that moment. The following is noted in the DSM-5 text:

> Such events occur on a continuum from brief visual or other sensory intrusions about part of the traumatic event without loss of reality orientation, to complete loss of awareness of present surroundings. These episodes, often referred to as "flashbacks," are typically brief but can be associated with prolonged distress and heightened arousal." (p. 275)

Because the term "flashbacks" has entered common parlance, the follow-up question specifically asks the patient whether he or she has experienced flashbacks of the event.

Criteria B4 and B5—Psychological distress or physiological reactions to internal or external cues. Responses to internal or external cues are separated into two PTSD items; Criterion B4 addresses intense or prolonged psychological distress, and Criterion B5 addresses marked physiological reactions. The SCID-5-CV introduces the assessment of these items with a single question that first establishes the cause-and-effect relationship between exposure to internal or external cues that symbolize or resemble the traumatic event and the development of an intense and unpleasant emotional or physical response. Internal cues can include physical sensations associated with the traumatic event. As noted in the DSM-5 text:

> The triggering cue could be a physical sensation (e.g., dizziness for survivors of head trauma; rapid heartbeat for a previously traumatized child), particularly for individuals with highly somatic presentations. (p. 275)

If the patient denies having any kind of reaction to reminders of the trauma, both Criterion B4 (psychological distress) and Criterion B5 (physiological reactions) can be rated "—". If the patient acknowledges having had some sort of reaction, then the clinician should inquire whether it was an intense or prolonged emotional reaction (item label G17) or a physical reaction (item label G18) and then rate each item accordingly.

Criterion C—Persistent avoidance of stimuli associated with the event. The diagnosis of PTSD requires persistent avoidance of stimuli associated with the traumatic event. In the context of this criterion, the DSM-5 text (p. 275) defines this persistence as "always or almost always" avoiding such stimuli, although without any specification of a minimum duration for this avoidance behavior in Criterion C. The SCID-5-CV has operationalized this requirement as requiring the avoidance to occur almost all of the time for more than 1 month, in keeping with the "more than 1 month" duration requirement in Criterion F. It is also important for the clinician to establish that this avoidance behavior began after the traumatic event occurred (i.e., avoidance associated with preexisting phobias should not count toward the diagnosis of PTSD).

Criterion C1—Avoidance of memories, thoughts, or feelings.   This item should be rated "+" if the patient makes deliberate efforts to avoid memories, thoughts, or feelings about or closely associated with the traumatic event. Because memories, thoughts, and feelings are internally generated, the only way to avoid them is to use distraction techniques such as keeping busy, playing computer or video games, watching TV, or using drugs or alcohol to "numb" oneself.

Criterion C2—Avoidance of external reminders that arouse distressing memories, thoughts, or feelings.   For this criterion, the person generally avoids external reminders of the traumatic event by going out of his or her way to avoid people, places, activities, objects, situations, or anything else likely to arouse memories, thoughts, or feelings about the event. For example, an individual who was involved in a serious car accident might persistently avoid driving, or a combat veteran might persistently avoid situations in which there are likely to be loud noises.

For some individuals, the need to make deliberate efforts to avoid external reminders may depend on the potential for encountering the reminder in his or her daily life. For example, consider an individual who lives in New York City and drives his car only when he needs to go to the supermarket. After getting into a serious car accident, he avoids driving his car to the supermarket and instead arranges for home delivery of his groceries. From a strict behavioral standpoint, his active avoidance behavior would not be persistent because he deliberately avoids driving only on those occasions when the need to drive arises. However, in the context of this criterion, persistent avoidance is as much attitudinal as behavioral. Even if the individual does not need to actively avoid a reminder every day as in this example, the avoidance would meet the persistent requirement if the person is persistently aware that he or she would not get into a car.

Criterion D—Negative alterations in cognitions and mood.   This cluster of Criterion D symptoms involves negative alterations in cognitions and mood that begin or worsen after the traumatic event occurred. The requirement that the symptoms begin or worsen after the traumatic event is especially important given both the relatively nontrauma-specific nature of several of these symptoms (e.g., persistent negative emotional state, diminished interest or participation in activities, inability to experience positive emotions) and the fact that some of these items (e.g., persistent and exaggerated negative beliefs or expectations about oneself, others, or the world) may represent preexisting personality traits.

Criterion D1—Inability to remember an important aspect of the event.   Given the common co-occurrence of trauma exposure with head trauma and with alcohol and substance use, it is important to ensure that the amnesia is not due to head injury and substance-induced memory loss (e.g., "blackouts") but is instead dissociative in nature.

Criterion D2—Negative beliefs or expectations about oneself, others, or the world. For this item to be rated "+", the patient's persistent and exaggerated negative beliefs about himself or herself, others, or the world should be associated with the traumatic event. This requirement is set forth in the first part of Criterion D (i.e., "Negative alterations in cognitions and mood associated with the traumatic event(s)"), which is established either by virtue of their content being somehow related to the traumatic event or by the fact that the beliefs developed only after exposure to the trauma. The DSM-5 criteria and text provide several examples of negative beliefs, such as "no one can be trusted," and "the world is completely dangerous." Developing the belief that the world is a completely dangerous place after exposure to a natural disaster or random act of violence suggests that the belief is associated with the trauma and would justify a rating of "+". Having a persistent belief that "no one can be trusted" is much less likely to be associated with those types of traumas and suggests that those beliefs were part of a preexisting belief system. (However, for other types of trauma, such as date or military rape, "no one can be trusted" may be a trauma-associated belief.) As with Criterion C, "persistent" is defined in DSM-5 as "always or almost always," which has been operationalized in the SCID-5-CV as "almost all of the time for more than 1 month."

Criterion D3—Persistent, distorted cognitions about the cause or consequences of the traumatic event.   This criterion requires the presence of persistent erroneous cognitions about the cause (i.e., who or what was to blame) or consequences (e.g., self-deprecation for having developed PTSD symptoms) of the traumatic event. Determining whether such cognitions are in fact erroneous can sometimes be challenging without firsthand knowledge about what actually happened. Although in some cases the cognitive distortions are obvious (e.g., "It's entirely my fault that my uncle abused me"), in other cases the distortions may be discernible only by virtue of the patient's unreasonable level of certainty about an ambiguous situation (e.g., a veteran insisting that he did not act quickly enough under fire as the primary cause for the rest of his platoon being attacked). As with Criterion D2, "persistent" is defined in DSM-5 as "always or almost always," which has been operationalized in the SCID-5-CV as "almost all of the time for more than 1 month."

Criterion D4—Persistent negative emotional state.   Although examples are provided in the criterion to illustrate the "negative emotional state" (i.e., "fear, horror, anger, guilt, or shame"), any negative emotional state would count, including feeling sad, empty, or numb. As with Criterion D2, "persistent" is defined in DSM-5 as "always or almost always," which has been operationalized as "almost all of the time for more than 1 month." Given that individuals with persistent negative mood states are at increased risk of developing PTSD when exposed to a traumatic event, it is important to discern that if the patient had a persistent negative emotional state before the trauma exposure, it significantly worsened after the trauma.

Criterion D5—Markedly diminished interest or participation in significant activities.
There are two components to this criterion (i.e., diminished interest in activities and diminished participation in activities), and the presence of either would justify a rating of "+". As with Criterion D4, it is especially important to ensure that the diminished

interest or participation in activities represents a change in the patient since his or her exposure to the traumatic event.

Criterion D6—*Feelings of detachment or estrangement from others.* This may be manifested as a general feeling of being disconnected from others or that the patient has closed himself or herself off from other people.

Criterion D7—*Persistent inability to experience positive emotions.* In contrast to the similar item in the DSM-IV PTSD criteria set (i.e., "restricted range of affect"), which suggested a general diminution in emotional responsiveness, only positive expressions of affect are restricted. As with Criterion D4, in Criterion D7 it is especially important to ensure that the inability to experience positive feelings represents a change in the patient since his or her exposure to the traumatic event.

Criterion E—Marked alterations in arousal and reactivity. At least two of the six listed items must have been present. It is important to establish that the marked alterations in arousal and reactivity are associated with the traumatic event by virtue of the fact that the symptoms began or worsened after the traumatic event occurred.

Criterion E1—*Irritable behavior and angry outbursts.* This item requires more than just irritable mood; a rating of "+" requires irritable behavior and angry outbursts that are typically manifested as verbal or physical aggression toward people or objects.

Criterion E2—*Reckless or self-destructive behavior.* According to the DSM-5 text (p. 275), examples of reckless or self-destructive behavior include dangerous driving, excessive alcohol or drug use, or self-injurious or suicidal behavior.

Criterion E3—*Hypervigilance.* The hypervigilance is manifested as a heightened sensitivity to potential threats, including those that are directly related to the traumatic experience (e.g., following a motor vehicle accident, being especially sensitive to the threat potentially caused by cars or trucks) and those not related to the traumatic event (e.g., being fearful of suffering a heart attack).

Criterion E4—*Exaggerated startle response.* This is manifested by the patient being very reactive to unexpected stimuli, such as loud noises or unexpected movements (e.g., being "jumpy" in response to a telephone ringing).

Criterion E5—*Problems with concentration.* This may be manifested by difficulty remembering daily events (e.g., forgetting one's telephone number) or attending to focused tasks (e.g., following a conversation for a sustained period of time).

Criterion E6—*Sleep disturbance.* Most commonly there are problems with sleep onset and maintenance.

Criterion F—Duration is more than 1 month. The minimum duration of symptoms in each of the symptom clusters (i.e., Criteria B, C, D, and E) is more than 1 month.

Criterion G—The disturbance causes clinically significant distress or impairment. The clinician starts by asking an open-ended question to determine the impact that the PTSD symptoms have had on the patient's life, as is done throughout the SCID-5-CV when assessing clinical significance. The additional follow-up questions are optional and cover various domains of functioning that might be impacted by PTSD symptoms. These questions should be asked only if it is not clear from the patient's previous answers whether the symptoms interfered with functioning.

Criterion H—Not due to a GMC and not substance/medication-induced. This item instructs the clinician to consider and rule out a GMC or a substance/medication as an etiological cause for the PTSD symptoms. Many individuals respond to trauma exposure by increasing their use of alcohol or other substances. Therefore, what may appear to be the symptoms of PTSD may in fact be due to the direct effects of alcohol or other substances.

10.10   Module H.   Attention-Deficit/Hyperactivity Disorder

10.10.1   Ratings for Current Adult Attention-Deficit/Hyperactivity Disorder (H1–H26)

The assessment for ADHD begins with two screening questions for Criterion A in item label H1 that are designed to determine whether or not to proceed with the full assessment of the 18 ADHD items: 1) "Over the past several years, have you been easily distracted or disorganized?" and 2) "Over the past several years, have you had a lot of difficulty sitting still or waiting your turn?" If the answer to both questions is "NO" and there is no evidence from the interview up to this point that the patient has had problems with inattention, hyperactivity, or impulsivity in the past 6 months, the clinician can skip out to Module I ("Screening for Other Current Disorders").

Criterion A1—Five out of nine inattention symptoms have persisted for at least 6 months. When the clinician inquires about each of the Criterion A1 inattention symptoms (item labels H2–H11), it is essential to first elicit examples of the behavior constituting the criterion and then ask additional follow-up questions to determine the extent to which the behavior "negatively impacts directly on social and academic/occupational activities" as required in the criterion. For example, if the patient answers "YES" to the initial question ("Have you often missed important details or made mistakes at work (or school) or while taking care of things at home?"), the clinician should then ask the patient to provide examples of this behavior. In some instances, the example will illustrate such an obvious negative impact on functioning that a rating of "+" is justified based on the example alone (e.g., "I made so many mistakes as a waitress getting customers' orders wrong that I got fired"). In other instances, where the potential negative impact of the behavior is less clear, additional follow-up questions (e.g., "How much did this affect your ability to do a good job at work?") may be required before a rating for the item can be given. Note that the SCID-5-CV is using the threshold of five out of nine items, which applies to "older adolescents and adults (age 17 and older)." If the patient is younger than age 17, the threshold of six out of nine items should be employed.

Criterion A2—Five out of nine hyperactive/impulsive symptoms have persisted for at least 6 months.   As for Criterion A1, it is imperative that the clinician obtain examples for Criterion A2 (item labels H12–H20) and determine whether the symptoms are sufficiently severe so as to have a direct negative impact on the patient's social and occupational/academic activities.

Criterion B—Several inattentive or hyperactive-impulsive symptoms were present before age 12.   ADHD is a neurodevelopmental disorder that has its onset during childhood. Therefore, as required in Criterion B, it is important to establish the presence of at least some of the Criterion A1 or Criterion A2 symptoms before age 12. If the patient has trouble remembering the age at which the symptoms that were coded "+" began, the SCID-5-CV provides a number of follow-up questions that inquire about problems during school that may be markers of the presence of ADHD symptoms (e.g., "Did teachers complain that you were not paying attention or that you talked too much in class? Were you ever sent to the principal's office because of your behavior? Did your parents complain that you were not able to sit still, that you were very messy, or that you were never ready on time?"). Given that adult recall of childhood symptoms tends to be unreliable, it is beneficial to obtain ancillary information if at all possible.

Criterion C—Symptoms are present in two or more settings.   It is important to establish that symptoms are present in more than one setting (e.g., not just at work).

Criterion D—Symptoms interfere with or reduce the quality of social, academic, or occupational functioning.   The clinician starts by asking an open-ended question to determine the impact that the ADHD symptoms have had on the patient's life. The follow-up questions are optional and cover various domains of functioning that might be impacted by the ADHD symptoms. They should be asked only if it is not clear from the patient's previous answers whether the symptoms interfered with or reduced the quality of social, academic, or occupational functioning.

Criterion E—The symptoms do not occur exclusively during the course of a psychotic disorder and are not better explained by another mental disorder.   Note that this exclusion has two components. If there is a comorbid psychotic disorder, ADHD cannot be diagnosed if the symptoms occur exclusively during the course of the psychotic disorder. In practical terms, this means that adult ADHD should be diagnosed only if the ADHD symptoms occurred in childhood, before the onset of the psychotic disorder. For other mental disorders, ADHD should not be diagnosed if the symptoms are better explained by the other mental disorder; this clinical judgment involves a consideration of whether the symptoms of inattention, hyperactivity, or impulsivity are best conceptualized as features of the other mental disorder.

Presentation specifiers for ADHD.   The diagnosis of ADHD is given according to the subtype that indicates the predominant presentation over the past 6 months: Combined

Presentation (if both Criterion A1 and Criterion A2 are met); Predominantly Inattentive Presentation (if Criterion A1 is met but not Criterion A2); or Predominantly Hyperactive/Impulsive Presentation (if Criterion A2 is met but not Criterion A1). The diagnostic codes for ADHD (included on the Diagnostic Summary Score Sheet) correspond to the choice of appropriate subtype.

10.11   Module I.   Screening for Other Current Disorders

As noted in the beginning of the SCID-5-CV User's Guide, the SCID-5-CV is a streamlined version of the SCID-5-RV, with fewer disorders assessed and all of the subtypes and specifiers (except for those that impact the diagnostic coding) omitted. Screening questions for most of the omitted disorders, taken verbatim from the SCID-5-RV, are provided in Module I to provide the clinician with the capability of screening for the possible presence of these disorders. Consequently, the time intervals for the application of these screening questions vary from 1 month up to 12 months, according to the applicable time frame in the SCID-5-RV. If the patient answers "YES" to a screening question, and the clinician is interested in whether or not the diagnostic criteria for the disorder are met, the clinician must refer to the DSM-5 diagnostic criteria and use his or her clinical assessment skills to make the diagnostic determination. To facilitate this effort, the DSM-5 diagnostic criteria for the screened disorders are included in Appendix A, "DSM-5 Criteria for Module I Disorders," of the SCID-5-CV User's Guide. Readers are referred to DSM-5 for full diagnostic criteria sets, including any omitted subtype and specifier descriptions, ICD-CM codes, coding notes, and recording procedures.

The disorders screened in Module I are in the sequence they appear in the SCID-5-RV, as follows (page numbers for DSM-5 criteria in parentheses):

Premenstrual Dysphoric Disorder (DSM-5 p. 171)
Specific Phobia (DSM-5 p. 197)
Separation Anxiety Disorder (DSM-5 p. 190)
Hoarding Disorder (DSM-5 p. 247)
Body Dysmorphic Disorder (DSM-5 p. 242)
Trichotillomania (Hair-Pulling Disorder) (DSM-5 p. 251)
Excoriation (Skin-Picking) Disorder (DSM-5 p. 254)
Insomnia Disorder (DSM-5 p. 362)
Hypersomnolence Disorder (DSM-5 p. 368)
Anorexia Nervosa (DSM-5 p. 338)
Bulimia Nervosa (DSM-5 p. 345)
Binge-Eating Disorder (DSM-5 p. 350)
Avoidant/Restrictive Food Intake Disorder (DSM-5 p. 334)
Somatic Symptom Disorder (DSM-5 p. 311)
Illness Anxiety Disorder (DSM-5 p. 315)
Intermittent Explosive Disorder (DSM-5 p. 466)
Gambling Disorder (DSM-5 p. 585)

10.12   Module J.   Adjustment Disorder

10.12.1   Ratings for Current Adjustment Disorder (J1–J5)

Adjustment Disorder applies to emotional or behavioral symptoms that 1) have developed in response to an identified psychosocial stressor and 2) do not meet criteria for another specific mental disorder (i.e., excluding the Other Specified and Unspecified categories). Consequently, Adjustment Disorder is placed at the very end of the SCID-5-CV, after evaluation of all of the other mental disorders in the SCID-5-CV has been completed. If the clinician has reached this point in the SCID-5-CV and there are symptoms that have occurred in the past 6 months that are not accounted for by any of the specific disorders already diagnosed in the SCID-5-CV (excluding Other Specified and Unspecified categories), then the clinician should proceed with the evaluation of Adjustment Disorder. The clinician is also given the option of recording on the Diagnostic Summary Score Sheet (page 4) the presence of other DSM-5 disorders not specifically covered in the SCID-5-CV; for example, Dissociative Identity Disorder or additional Other Specified and Unspecified Disorder categories (e.g., Other Specified or Unspecified Anxiety Disorder).

Criterion A—Development of symptoms in response to identifiable stressor. This criterion establishes that symptoms that are diagnostically unaccounted for and that led the clinician to commence the assessment of Adjustment Disorder have developed in response to a stressor. The first question determines whether the stressor was present before the onset of the symptoms. The second question ("IF YES") tries to establish whether the symptoms occurred in response to the stressor: "Do you think that (STRESSOR) had anything to do with your developing (SXS)?" The final question determines whether the onset of the symptoms has occurred within 3 months of the stressor. For single-event stressors, the focus is on how long it took after the stressor for the symptoms to develop. For chronic stressors that may be ongoing and without a clear end point, the focus is on when the chronic stressor started.

Criterion B—Marked distress that is out of proportion to the severity of stressor or clinically significant impairment in functioning.   This criterion requires either that the patient's distressing symptoms are out of proportion to the severity of the stressors (Criterion B1) or that the symptoms cause clinically significant distress or impairment (Criterion B2). Given the difficulty in determining whether the symptoms are more severe than they should be (i.e., out of proportion to the stressor), the order of the questions corresponding to the Criterion B subcomponents has been switched so that the assessment of impairment (Criterion B2) comes first; the clinician only needs to assess the proportionality of the symptoms (Criterion B1) if there is no clinically significant impairment in functioning.

Criterion C—Does not meet criteria for another mental disorder and is not an exacerbation of a preexisting mental disorder.   The two parenthetical questions in item label J3 are geared to assist the clinician with the assessment of the second part of

Criterion C, which excludes exacerbations of preexisting disorders. The first part of Criterion C should automatically be true (i.e., criteria have not been met for another DSM-5 mental disorder) because of the SCID-5-CV requirement for this to be true before proceeding with the evaluation of current Adjustment Disorder.

Criterion D—Does not represent normal bereavement. Because bereavement can manifest as a clinically significant symptomatic reaction to a stressor (i.e., loss of a loved one), this criterion is needed to prevent normal grief from being pathologized.

Criterion E—Symptoms do not persist for more than 6 months after the stressor or its consequences have terminated. There appears to be a strict upper limit of 6 months for the duration of symptoms after the stressor or its consequences have terminated for the presentation to be considered consistent with a diagnosis of Adjustment Disorder. However, the vagueness of the concept of the "consequences" of the stressor effectively means that there is no time limit for many (if not most) stressors.

Adjustment Disorder subtypes. The diagnosis of Adjustment Disorder is given according to the subtype that indicates the predominant symptoms characterizing the response to the stressor. The diagnostic codes for Adjustment Disorder (included on the Diagnostic Summary Score Sheet) correspond to the choice of appropriate subtype.

11.   Training

Refer to the SCID Web site (www.scid5.org) for the most up-to-date information regarding available training materials; new materials are continually being developed.
   Ideally, training should involve the following sequence:

1. Study Sections 5–8 in this User's Guide, which respectively cover the SCID-5-CV basic features, administration, conventions and usage, and do's and don'ts.
2. Carefully read through every word of the sections of the SCID-5-CV that you are planning to use, making sure that you understand all of the instructions, the questions, and the DSM-5 diagnostic criteria. As you are reading through each module, refer to the corresponding instructions for that module in Section 10, "Special Instructions for Individual Modules," in the User's Guide. Review the DSM-5 text sections "Diagnostic Features" and "Differential Diagnosis" for those disorders included in the SCID-5-CV.
3. Now practice reading the SCID-5-CV questions aloud so that eventually it sounds as if SCID is your mother tongue.
4. Try out the SCID-5-CV with a colleague (or significant other) who can assume the role of a patient. Have them portray a case of someone they know.
5. Watch the didactic video training program SCID-101. Please refer to the SCID Web site (www.scid5.org) for information about the contents of the didactic videos and how to order them.

6. Role-play the cases in Appendix B, "Training Materials," with a colleague. These cases have been designed to take you through the SCID-5-CV modules, not necessarily to demonstrate your dramatic talent.

7. Watch videos of SCID-5-CV interviews (which can be ordered from the SCID Web site, www.scid5.org) and make your own ratings as the interviews proceed. Compare your ratings with the "expert" ratings that are included with each video.

8. Try out the SCID-5-CV on actual patients with other clinicians who are learning how to use the SCID-5-CV as observers making independent ratings during the interview. This should be followed by a discussion of the interviewing technique and sources of disagreement in the ratings.

9. Consider setting up an on-site SCID-5-CV training workshop conducted by an associate of the Biometrics Research Department (e-mail: scid5@columbia.edu). On-site SCID training consists primarily of a demonstration of a live SCID interview followed by group supervision of SCID interviews conducted by the trainees on actual patients. It is expected that the trainees will have watched the SCID-101 didactic training series before the on-site training so that they are prepared to participate in the group interviews. The training usually begins with a discussion of any issues that have arisen during the didactic portion of the training, followed by a series of SCID interviews conducted on volunteer patients. Typically the first SCID interview is conducted by the trainer in order to demonstrate his or her SCID technique, followed by interviews conducted by the trainees (one or two trainees per interview, depending on the number of people being trained and the duration of the training).

10. Another way to insure that the SCID trainees are administering the SCID properly is to record the trainees and then send the recordings (plus the accompanying rated SCIDs) to Biometrics Research for review and critique. Refer to the SCID Web site for more information about how to use this service and its costs.

12.   Psychometric Issues

12.1   SCID Reliability

Reliability for diagnostic assessment instruments is generally evaluated by comparing the agreement between independent evaluations by two or more interviewers across a group of subjects. The results for categorical constructs, such as the DSM diagnoses being assessed by the SCID, are usually reported with a statistic called kappa that takes into account agreement due to chance (Spitzer et al. 1967). Kappa values above .70 are considered to reflect good agreement; values from .50 to .70, fair agreement; and below .50, poor agreement (Landis and Koch 1977). Because the SCID is a not a fully structured interview, and requires the clinical judgment of the interviewer, the reliability of the SCID is very much a function of the particular circumstances in which it is being used.

Table 12–1 provides a summary of selected published reliability studies of previous SCID versions. (Refer to the SCID Web site for the most up-to-date list of SCID reliability studies, including the reliability of the SCID-5 as it becomes available). Three studies have examined the reliability of the SCID for DSM-IV. Lobbestael and colleagues (2011) examined the reliability of the Dutch version of the SCID. In a mixed sample of 151 inpatients and outpatients during a joint reliability study, the first rater recorded his or her SCID interview, which was then rated by a second interviewer blind to the first rater's scores and diagnoses. Zanarini and colleagues (2000) examined both joint and test-retest reliability of the SCID as part of the Collaborative Longitudinal Personality Disorders Study. In their study, 84 pairs of raters viewed videotaped SCID interviews for the joint interrater component, and interviewers conducted independent interviews on 52 subjects 7–10 days apart for the test-retest component. Martin and colleagues (2000) examined the reliability of alcohol and other substance use disorders in 71 adolescents using a joint interrater design (two interviewers made independent ratings during the same live SCID interview).

Zanarini and Frankenburg (2001) examined the reliability of the SCID for DSM-III-R using four different methods: interrater reliability of 45 inpatients using conjoint interviews, test-retest reliability of 30 subjects with a 7–10 day time interval between interviews, interrater reliability of 48 patients at their 2- or 4-year follow-up assessment using conjoint interviews, and interrater reliability at time of longitudinal follow-up using 36 audiotaped interviews that were made during the initial evaluation phase. In the most extensive reliability study of the SCID for DSM-III-R, Williams and colleagues (1992) examined multisite test-retest reliability in 592 patients who were a mixture of inpatients, outpatients, patients with substance use issues, and patients selected from the community. Skre and colleagues (1991) determined the interrater reliability of the SCID for DSM-III-R by having three raters independently rate 54 audiotaped SCID interviews.

As can be seen immediately in Table 12–1, the range of kappa values from different studies and for different diagnoses is enormous. Many factors influence the reliability of an interview instrument such as the SCID. We will address some of these in the following discussion.

12.1.1   Joint Interviews Versus Test-Retest Design

In some studies, a subject is interviewed by one clinician while others observe (either in person or by reviewing a tape) and then make independent ratings ("joint"). Joint interviews produce the highest reliability because all raters are hearing exactly the same story, and because the trail of skip instructions provides clues to the observers about the ratings made by the interviewer. A more stringent test of reliability (test-retest, also called reliability based on independent interviews) entails having the same subject interviewed at two different times by two different interviewers. This method tends to lead to lower levels of reliability because the subject may, even when prompted with the same questions, tell different stories to the two interviewers ("information variance"), resulting in divergent ratings.

TABLE 12–1.　Selected SCID-I[a] reliability studies

Reference	Lobbestael et al. 2011	Zanarini et al. 2000	Zanarini et al. 2000	Martin et al. 2000	Zanarini and Frankenburg 2001	Zanarini and Frankenburg 2001	Zanarini and Frankenburg 2001	Zanarini and Frankenburg 2001	Williams et al. 1992	Skre et al. 1991
Population studied	N=151 (mixed inpt./outpt.)	N=27 (videotape sample)	N=52 (test-retest sample)	N=71 (outpt. adolescent alcohol users)	N=30	N=45 (inpt.)	N=48	N=30	N=592; (mixed inpt., outpt., nonpt.)	N=54
Version of SCID	DSM-IV	DSM-IV	DSM-IV	DSM-IV	DSM-III-R	DSM-III-R	DSM-III-R	DSM-III-R	DSM-III-R	DSM-III-R
Design of reliability study	Joint; audiotape	Joint; 84 rater-pairs from 4 sites	7–10 day interval test-retest	Joint; observed live	7–10 day interval test-retest	Joint; observed live	Joint; observed live	Joint; audiotape	1–3 week interval test-retest	Joint; audiotape
Major Depressive Disorder	.66	.80	.61		.73	.90	.93	1.0	.64	.93
Dysthymic Disorder	.81	.76	.35		.60	.91	.93	.84	.40	.88
Bipolar Disorder									.84	.79
Schizophrenia									.65	.94
Alcohol Dependence/Abuse	.65	1.0	.77	.94	.77	1.0			.75	.96
Other Substance Dependence/Abuse	.77	1.0	.76	.94	.82	.95			.84	.85
Panic Disorder	.67	.65	.65		.82	.88			.58	.88
Social Phobia	.83	.63	.59		.53	.86	.71	1.0	.47	.72
Obsessive-Compulsive Disorder	.65	.57	.60		.42	.70			.59	.40
Generalized Anxiety Disorder	.75	.63	.44		.63	.73			.56	.95
Posttraumatic Stress Disorder	.77	.88	.78		1.0	1.0	1.0	1.0		.77
Any Somatoform Disorder										–.03
Any Eating Disorder	.61	.77	.64							
Agoraphobia	.60									
Specific Phobia	.83									

[a]SCID-I=Structured Clinical Interview for DSM Axis I Disorders.

12.1.2 Interviewer Training

Raters who are well trained, and particularly, raters who train and work together are likely to have better agreement on ratings. It is worth noting that the professional discipline of the interviewer (e.g., psychiatrist, psychologist, social worker) does not appear to contribute to differences in reliability.

12.1.3 Subject Population

Subjects with the most severe and florid psychiatric disorders (e.g., patients repeatedly hospitalized with Schizophrenia or Bipolar Disorder) are likely to yield more reliable SCID diagnoses than subjects with milder psychiatric conditions that border on normality. This reflects the fact that relatively minor diagnostic disagreements are more likely to have a profound effect when the severity of the disorder is just at the diagnostic threshold. For example, a disagreement about a single criterion for a subject with exactly five out of nine symptoms of a Major Depressive Episode can make the difference between having a diagnosis of Major Depressive Disorder or Other Specified Depressive Disorder, whereas a one-item disagreement for a subject with seven out of nine items would probably not result in any apparent disagreement on the diagnosis.

12.1.4 Disorder Base Rates

The base rates of the diagnoses in the population being studied affect the reported reliability. If the error of measurement for a diagnostic instrument is constant, reliability varies directly with the base rates. It is thus harder to obtain good reliability for a rare diagnosis than for a common diagnosis. For example, SCID reliability for Major Depressive Disorder will be higher in a mood disorders clinic than in a community sample, in which the base rate of Major Depressive Disorder is much lower.

12.2 SCID Validity

The validity of a diagnostic assessment technique is generally measured by determining the agreement between the diagnoses made by the assessment technique and some hypothetical "gold standard." Unfortunately, a gold standard for psychiatric diagnosis remains elusive. There is obvious difficulty in using ordinary clinical diagnoses as the standard because structured interviews have been specifically designed to improve on the inherent limitations of an unstructured clinical interview. In fact, a number of studies have used the SCID as the gold standard in determining the accuracy of clinical diagnoses (Fennig et al. 1994a; Kashner et al. 2003; Ramirez Basco et al. 2000; Shear et al. 2000; Steiner et al. 1995).

Perhaps the most accepted (albeit flawed) standard used in psychiatric diagnostic studies is known as a "best estimate diagnosis." Spitzer proposed an operationalization of this best estimate diagnosis, which he termed the "LEAD standard" (Spitzer 1983). This standard involves conducting a longitudinal assessment (L) (i.e., relying on data collected over time), done by expert diagnosticians (E), using all data (AD) that are available about the subjects, such as family informants, review of medical records, and observations of clinical staff. Although conceptually the LEAD standard is appealing, the difficulty in implementing it accounts for its limited use. Several studies (Fennig et al. 1994b, 1996; Kranzler et al. 1995, 1996; Ramirez Basco et al. 2000) used approximations of the LEAD procedure. Both demonstrated superior validity of the SCID over standard clinical interviews at intake episode.

References

American Psychiatric Association: Diagnostic and Statistical Manual of Mental Disorders, 3rd Edition. Washington, DC, American Psychiatric Association, 1980

American Psychiatric Association: Diagnostic and Statistical Manual of Mental Disorders, 3rd Edition, Revised. Washington, DC, American Psychiatric Association, 1987

American Psychiatric Association: Diagnostic and Statistical Manual of Mental Disorders, 4th Edition. Washington, DC, American Psychiatric Association, 1994

American Psychiatric Association: Diagnostic and Statistical Manual of Mental Disorders, 4th Edition, Text Revision. Washington, DC, American Psychiatric Association, 2000

American Psychiatric Association: Diagnostic and Statistical Manual of Mental Disorders, 5th Edition. Arlington, VA, American Psychiatric Association, 2013

Endicott J, Spitzer, RL: A diagnostic interview: the schedule for affective disorders and schizophrenia. Arch Gen Psych 35(7):837–844, 1978

Feighner JP, Robins E, Guze SB, et al: Diagnostic criteria for use in psychiatric research. Arch Gen Psychiatry 26(1):57–63, 1972

Fennig S, Craig T, Lavelle J, et al: Best-estimate versus structured interview-based diagnosis in first-admission psychosis. Compr Psychiatry 35(5):341–348, 1994a

Fennig S, Craig T, Tanenberg-Karant M, Bromet EJ: Comparison of facility and research diagnoses in first-admission psychotic patients. Am J Psychiatry 151(10):1423–1429, 1994b

Fennig S, Naisberg-Fennig S, Craig TJ, et al: Comparison of clinical and research diagnoses of substance use disorders in a first-admission psychotic sample. Am J Addict 5(1):40–48, 1996

First MB: DSM-5 Handbook of Differential Diagnosis. Washington, DC, American Psychiatric Publishing, 2014

Helzer JE, Robins LN, Croughan JL, Welner A: Renard diagnostic interview. Its reliability and procedural validity with physicians and lay interviewers. Arch Gen Psych 38(4):393–398, 1981

Kashner TM, Rush AJ, Suris A, et al: Impact of structured clinical interviews on physicians' practices in community mental health settings. Psychiatr Serv 54(5):712–718, 2003

Kranzler HR, Kadden RM, Burleson JA, et al: Validity of psychiatric diagnoses in patients with substance use disorders: is the interview more important than the interviewer? Compr Psychiatry 36(4):278–288, 1995

Kranzler HR, Kadden RM, Babor TF, et al: Validity of the SCID in substance abuse patients. Addiction 91(6):859–868, 1996

Landis JR, Koch GG: The measurement of observer agreement for categorical data. Biometrics 33(1):159–174, 1977

Lobbestael J, Leurgans M, Arntz A: Interrater reliability of the Structured Clinical Interview for DSM-IV Axis I Disorders (SCID I) and Axis II Disorders (SCID II). Clin Psychol Psychother 18(1):75–79, 2011

Martin CS, Pollock NK, Bukstein OG, Lynch KG: Interrater reliability of the SCID alcohol and substance use disorders section among adolescents. Drug and Alcohol Depend 59(2):173–176, 2000

Ramirez Basco M, Bostic JQ, Davies D, et al: Methods to improve diagnostic accuracy in a community mental health setting. Am J Psychiatry 157(10):1599–1605, 2000

Shear MK, Greeno C, Kang K, et al: Diagnosis of nonpsychotic patients in community clinics. Am J Psychiatry 157(4):581–587, 2000

Shore, JH, Savin D, Orton H, et al: Diagnostic reliability of telepsychiatry in American Indian veterans. Am J Psychiatry 164(1):115–118, 2007

Skre I, Onstad S, Torgersen S, Kringlen E: High interrater reliability for the Structured Clinical Interview for DSM-III-R Axis I (SCID-I). Acta Psychiatr Scand 84(2):167–173, 1991

Spitzer RL: Psychiatric diagnosis: are clinicians still necessary? Compr Psychiatry 24(5):399–411, 1983

Spitzer RL, Cohen J, Fleiss JL, Endicott J: Quantification of agreement in psychiatric diagnosis. A new approach. Arch Gen Psych 17(1):83–87, 1967

Spitzer R, Endicott J, Robins E: Research diagnostic criteria: rationale and reliability. Arch Gen Psychiatry 35:773–782, 1978

Spitzer RL, Williams JBW, Gibbon M, First MB: Structured Clinical Interview for DSM-III-R, Patient Edition/Nonpatient Edition (SCID-P/SCID-NP). Washington, DC, American Psychiatric Press, 1990a

Spitzer RL, Williams JBW, Gibbon M, First MB: Structured Clinician Interview for DSM-III-R Axis II Disorders (SCID-II). Washington, DC, American Psychiatric Press, 1990b

Spitzer RL, Williams JB, Gibbon M, First MB: The Structured Clinical Interview for DSM-III-R (SCID). I: History, rationale, and description. Arch Gen Psychiatry 49(8):624–629, 1992

Spitzer RL, Gibbon M, Skodol AE, et al: DSM-IV-TR Casebook: A Learning Companion to the Diagnostic and Statistical Manual of Mental Disorders, Fourth Edition, Text Revision. Washington, DC, American Psychiatric Publishing, 2002

Steiner JL, Tebes JK, Sledge WH, Waler ML: A comparison of the structured clinical interview for DSM-III-R and clinical diagnoses. J Nerv Ment Dis 183(6):365–369, 1995

Williams JB, Gibbon M, First MB, Spitzer RL, et al: The Structured Clinical Interview for DSM-III-R (SCID) II. Multisite test-retest reliability. Arch Gen Psychiatry 49(8):630–636, 1992

Zanarini MC, Frankenburg FR: Attainment and maintenance of reliability of Axis I and Axis II disorders over the course of a longitudinal study. Compr Psychiatry 42(5):369–374, 2001

Zanarini MC, Skodol AE, Bender D, et al: The Collaborative Longitudinal Personality Disorders Study: reliability of Axis I and II diagnoses. J Pers Disord 14(4):291–299, 2000

DSM-5 Criteria for Module I Disorders

Premenstrual Dysphoric Disorder

A. In the majority of menstrual cycles, at least five symptoms must be present in the final week before the onset of menses, start to *improve* within a few days after the onset of menses, and become *minimal* or absent in the week postmenses.

B. One (or more) of the following symptoms must be present:

1. Marked affective lability (e.g., mood swings; feeling suddenly sad or tearful, or increased sensitivity to rejection).
2. Marked irritability or anger or increased interpersonal conflicts.
3. Marked depressed mood, feelings of hopelessness, or self-deprecating thoughts.
4. Marked anxiety, tension, and/or feelings of being keyed up or on edge.

C. One (or more) of the following symptoms must additionally be present, to reach a total of *five* symptoms when combined with symptoms from Criterion B above.

1. Decreased interest in usual activities (e.g., work, school, friends, hobbies).
2. Subjective difficulty in concentration.
3. Lethargy, easy fatigability, or marked lack of energy.
4. Marked change in appetite; overeating; or specific food cravings.
5. Hypersomnia or insomnia.
6. A sense of being overwhelmed or out of control.
7. Physical symptoms such as breast tenderness or swelling, joint or muscle pain, a sensation of "bloating," or weight gain.

Note: The symptoms in Criteria A–C must have been met for most menstrual cycles that occurred in the preceding year.

D. The symptoms are associated with clinically significant distress or interference with work, school, usual social activities, or relationships with others (e.g., avoidance of social activities; decreased productivity and efficiency at work, school, or home).

E. The disturbance is not merely an exacerbation of the symptoms of another disorder, such as major depressive disorder, panic disorder, persistent depressive disorder (dysthymia), or a personality disorder (although it may co-occur with any of these disorders).

F. Criterion A should be confirmed by prospective daily ratings during at least two symptomatic cycles. (**Note:** The diagnosis may be made provisionally prior to this confirmation.)

G. The symptoms are not attributable to the physiological effects of a substance (e.g., a drug of abuse, a medication, other treatment) or another medical condition (e.g., hyperthyroidism).

Specific Phobia

A. Marked fear or anxiety about a specific object or situation (e.g., flying, heights, animals, receiving an injection, seeing blood).

   Note: In children, the fear or anxiety may be expressed by crying, tantrums, freezing, or clinging.

B. The phobic object or situation almost always provokes immediate fear or anxiety.

C. The phobic object or situation is actively avoided or endured with intense fear or anxiety.

D. The fear or anxiety is out of proportion to the actual danger posed by the specific object or situation and to the sociocultural context.

E. The fear, anxiety, or avoidance is persistent, typically lasting for 6 months or more.

F. The fear, anxiety, or avoidance causes clinically significant distress or impairment in social, occupational, or other important areas of functioning.

G. The disturbance is not better explained by the symptoms of another mental disorder, including fear, anxiety, and avoidance of situations associated with panic-like symptoms or other incapacitating symptoms (as in agoraphobia); objects or situations related to obsessions (as in obsessive-compulsive disorder); reminders of traumatic events (as in posttraumatic stress disorder); separation from home or attachment figures (as in separation anxiety disorder); or social situations (as in social anxiety disorder).

Specify if:

Animal (e.g., spiders, insects, dogs).

Natural environment (e.g., heights, storms, water).

Blood-injection-injury (e.g., needles, invasive medical procedures).

Situational (e.g., airplanes, elevators, enclosed places).

Other (e.g., situations that may lead to choking or vomiting; in children, e.g., loud sounds or costumed characters).

Separation Anxiety Disorder

A. Developmentally inappropriate and excessive fear or anxiety concerning separation from those to whom the individual is attached, as evidenced by at least three of the following:

1. Recurrent excessive distress when anticipating or experiencing separation from home or from major attachment figures.
2. Persistent and excessive worry about losing major attachment figures or about possible harm to them, such as illness, injury, disasters, or death.
3. Persistent and excessive worry about experiencing an untoward event (e.g., getting lost, being kidnapped, having an accident, becoming ill) that causes separation from a major attachment figure.
4. Persistent reluctance or refusal to go out, away from home, to school, to work, or elsewhere because of fear of separation.
5. Persistent and excessive fear of or reluctance about being alone or without major attachment figures at home or in other settings.
6. Persistent reluctance or refusal to sleep away from home or to go to sleep without being near a major attachment figure.
7. Repeated nightmares involving the theme of separation.
8. Repeated complaints of physical symptoms (e.g., headaches, stomachaches, nausea, vomiting) when separation from major attachment figures occurs or is anticipated.

B. The fear, anxiety, or avoidance is persistent, lasting at least 4 weeks in children and adolescents and typically 6 months or more in adults.

C. The disturbance causes clinically significant distress or impairment in social, academic, occupational, or other important areas of functioning.

D. The disturbance is not better explained by another mental disorder, such as refusing to leave home because of excessive resistance to change in autism spectrum disorder; delusions or hallucinations concerning separation in psychotic disorders; refusal to go outside without a trusted companion in agoraphobia; worries about ill health or other harm befalling significant others in generalized anxiety disorder; or concerns about having an illness in illness anxiety disorder.

Hoarding Disorder

A. Persistent difficulty discarding or parting with possessions, regardless of their actual value.

B. This difficulty is due to a perceived need to save the items and to distress associated with discarding them.

C. The difficulty discarding possessions results in the accumulation of possessions that congest and clutter active living areas and substantially compromises their intended use. If living areas are uncluttered, it is only because of the interventions of third parties (e.g., family members, cleaners, authorities).

D. The hoarding causes clinically significant distress or impairment in social, occupational, or other important areas of functioning (including maintaining a safe environment for self and others).

E. The hoarding is not attributable to another medical condition (e.g., brain injury, cerebrovascular disease, Prader-Willi syndrome).

F. The hoarding is not better explained by the symptoms of another mental disorder (e.g., obsessions in obsessive-compulsive disorder, decreased energy in major depressive disorder, delusions in schizophrenia or another psychotic disorder, cognitive deficits in major neurocognitive disorder, restricted interests in autism spectrum disorder).

Body Dysmorphic Disorder

A. Preoccupation with one or more perceived defects or flaws in physical appearance that are not observable or appear slight to others.

B. At some point during the course of the disorder, the individual has performed repetitive behaviors (e.g., mirror checking, excessive grooming, skin picking, reassurance seeking) or mental acts (e.g., comparing his or her appearance with that of others) in response to the appearance concerns.

C. The preoccupation causes clinically significant distress or impairment in social, occupational, or other important areas of functioning.

D. The appearance preoccupation is not better explained by concerns with body fat or weight in an individual whose symptoms meet diagnostic criteria for an eating disorder.

Trichotillomania (Hair-Pulling Disorder)

A. Recurrent pulling out of one's hair, resulting in hair loss.

B. Repeated attempts to decrease or stop hair pulling.

C. The hair pulling causes clinically significant distress or impairment in social, occupational, or other important areas of functioning.

D. The hair pulling or hair loss is not attributable to another medical condition (e.g., a dermatological condition).

E. The hair pulling is not better explained by the symptoms of another mental disorder (e.g., attempts to improve a perceived defect or flaw in appearance in body dysmorphic disorder).

Excoriation (Skin-Picking) Disorder

A. Recurrent skin picking resulting in skin lesions.

B. Repeated attempts to decrease or stop skin picking.

C. The skin picking causes clinically significant distress or impairment in social, occupational, or other important areas of functioning.

D. The skin picking is not attributable to the physiological effects of a substance (e.g., cocaine) or another medical condition (e.g., scabies).

E. The skin picking is not better explained by symptoms of another mental disorder (e.g., delusions or tactile hallucinations in a psychotic disorder, attempts to improve a perceived defect or flaw in appearance in body dysmorphic disorder, stereotypies in stereotypic movement disorder, or intention to harm oneself in nonsuicidal self-injury).

Insomnia Disorder

A. A predominant complaint of dissatisfaction with sleep quantity or quality, associated with one (or more) of the following symptoms:

1. Difficulty initiating sleep. (In children, this may manifest as difficulty initiating sleep without caregiver intervention.)
2. Difficulty maintaining sleep, characterized by frequent awakenings or problems returning to sleep after awakenings. (In children, this may manifest as difficulty returning to sleep without caregiver intervention.)
3. Early-morning awakening with inability to return to sleep.

B. The sleep disturbance causes clinically significant distress or impairment in social, occupational, educational, academic, behavioral, or other important areas of functioning.
C. The sleep difficulty occurs at least 3 nights per week.
D. The sleep difficulty is present for at least 3 months.
E. The sleep difficulty occurs despite adequate opportunity for sleep.
F. The insomnia is not better explained by and does not occur exclusively during the course of another sleep-wake disorder (e.g., narcolepsy, a breathing-related sleep disorder, a circadian rhythm sleep-wake disorder, a parasomnia).
G. The insomnia is not attributable to the physiological effects of a substance (e.g., a drug of abuse, a medication).
H. Coexisting mental disorders and medical conditions do not adequately explain the predominant complaint of insomnia.

Hypersomnolence Disorder

A. Self-reported excessive sleepiness (hypersomnolence) despite a main sleep period lasting at least 7 hours, with at least one of the following symptoms:

1. Recurrent periods of sleep or lapses into sleep within the same day.
2. A prolonged main sleep episode of more than 9 hours per day that is nonrestorative (i.e., unrefreshing).
3. Difficulty being fully awake after abrupt awakening.

B. The hypersomnolence occurs at least three times per week, for at least 3 months.
C. The hypersomnolence is accompanied by significant distress or impairment in cognitive, social, occupational, or other important areas of functioning.
D. The hypersomnolence is not better explained by and does not occur exclusively during the course of another sleep disorder (e.g., narcolepsy, breathing-related sleep disorder, circadian rhythm sleep-wake disorder, or a parasomnia).
E. The hypersomnolence is not attributable to the physiological effects of a substance (e.g., a drug of abuse, a medication).
F. Coexisting mental and medical disorders do not adequately explain the predominant complaint of hypersomnolence.

Anorexia Nervosa

A. Restriction of energy intake relative to requirements, leading to a significantly low body weight in the context of age, sex, developmental trajectory, and physical health. *Significantly low weight* is defined as a weight that is less than minimally normal or, for children and adolescents, less than that minimally expected.

B. Intense fear of gaining weight or of becoming fat, or persistent behavior that interferes with weight gain, even though at a significantly low weight.

C. Disturbance in the way in which one's body weight or shape is experienced, undue influence of body weight or shape on self-evaluation, or persistent lack of recognition of the seriousness of the current low body weight.

Specify whether:

Restricting type: During the last 3 months, the individual has not engaged in recurrent episodes of binge eating or purging behavior (i.e., self-induced vomiting or the misuse of laxatives, diuretics, or enemas). This subtype describes presentations in which weight loss is accomplished primarily through dieting, fasting, and/or excessive exercise.

Binge-eating/purging type: During the last 3 months, the individual has engaged in recurrent episodes of binge eating or purging behavior (i.e., self-induced vomiting or the misuse of laxatives, diuretics, or enemas).

Bulimia Nervosa

A. Recurrent episodes of binge eating. An episode of binge eating is characterized by both of the following:

1. Eating, in a discrete period of time (e.g., within any 2-hour period), an amount of food that is definitely larger than what most individuals would eat in a similar period of time under similar circumstances.

2. A sense of lack of control over eating during the episode (e.g., a feeling that one cannot stop eating or control what or how much one is eating).

B. Recurrent inappropriate compensatory behaviors in order to prevent weight gain, such as self-induced vomiting; misuse of laxatives, diuretics, or other medications; fasting; or excessive exercise.

C. The binge eating and inappropriate compensatory behaviors both occur, on average, at least once a week for 3 months.

D. Self-evaluation is unduly influenced by body shape and weight.

E. The disturbance does not occur exclusively during episodes of anorexia nervosa.

Binge-Eating Disorder

A. Recurrent episodes of binge eating. An episode of binge eating is characterized by both of the following:

1. Eating, in a discrete period of time (e.g., within any 2-hour period), an amount of food that is definitely larger than what most people would eat in a similar period of time under similar circumstances.
2. A sense of lack of control over eating during the episode (e.g., a feeling that one cannot stop eating or control what or how much one is eating).

B. The binge-eating episodes are associated with three (or more) of the following:

1. Eating much more rapidly than normal.
2. Eating until feeling uncomfortably full.
3. Eating large amounts of food when not feeling physically hungry.
4. Eating alone because of feeling embarrassed by how much one is eating.
5. Feeling disgusted with oneself, depressed, or very guilty afterward.

C. Marked distress regarding binge eating is present.
D. The binge eating occurs, on average, at least once a week for 3 months.
E. The binge eating is not associated with the recurrent use of inappropriate compensatory behavior as in bulimia nervosa and does not occur exclusively during the course of bulimia nervosa or anorexia nervosa.

Avoidant/Restrictive Food Intake Disorder

A. An eating or feeding disturbance (e.g., apparent lack of interest in eating or food; avoidance based on the sensory characteristics of food; concern about aversive consequences of eating) as manifested by persistent failure to meet appropriate nutritional and/or energy needs associated with one (or more) of the following:

1. Significant weight loss (or failure to achieve expected weight gain or faltering growth in children).
2. Significant nutritional deficiency.
3. Dependence on enteral feeding or oral nutritional supplements.
4. Marked interference with psychosocial functioning.

B. The disturbance is not better explained by lack of available food or by an associated culturally sanctioned practice.
C. The eating disturbance does not occur exclusively during the course of anorexia nervosa or bulimia nervosa, and there is no evidence of a disturbance in the way in which one's body weight or shape is experienced.
D. The eating disturbance is not attributable to a concurrent medical condition or not better explained by another mental disorder. When the eating disturbance occurs in the context of another condition or disorder, the severity of the eating disturbance exceeds that routinely associated with the condition or disorder and warrants additional clinical attention.

Somatic Symptom Disorder

A. One or more somatic symptoms that are distressing or result in significant disruption of daily life.

B. Excessive thoughts, feelings, or behaviors related to the somatic symptoms or associated health concerns as manifested by at least one of the following:

1. Disproportionate and persistent thoughts about the seriousness of one's symptoms.
2. Persistently high level of anxiety about health or symptoms.
3. Excessive time and energy devoted to these symptoms or health concerns.

C. Although any one somatic symptom may not be continuously present, the state of being symptomatic is persistent (typically more than 6 months).

Illness Anxiety Disorder

A. Preoccupation with having or acquiring a serious illness.

B. Somatic symptoms are not present or, if present, are only mild in intensity. If another medical condition is present or there is a high risk for developing a medical condition (e.g., strong family history is present), the preoccupation is clearly excessive or disproportionate.

C. There is a high level of anxiety about health, and the individual is easily alarmed about personal health status.

D. The individual performs excessive health-related behaviors (e.g., repeatedly checks his or her body for signs of illness) or exhibits maladaptive avoidance (e.g., avoids doctor appointments and hospitals).

E. Illness preoccupation has been present for at least 6 months, but the specific illness that is feared may change over that period of time.

F. The illness-related preoccupation is not better explained by another mental disorder, such as somatic symptom disorder, panic disorder, generalized anxiety disorder, body dysmorphic disorder, obsessive-compulsive disorder, or delusional disorder, somatic type.

Intermittent Explosive Disorder

A. Recurrent behavioral outbursts representing a failure to control aggressive impulses as manifested by either of the following:

   1. Verbal aggression (e.g., temper tantrums, tirades, verbal arguments or fights) or physical aggression toward property, animals, or other individuals, occurring twice weekly, on average, for a period of 3 months. The physical aggression does not result in damage or destruction of property and does not result in physical injury to animals or other individuals.

   2. Three behavioral outbursts involving damage or destruction of property and/ or physical assault involving physical injury against animals or other individuals occurring within a 12-month period.

B. The magnitude of aggressiveness expressed during the recurrent outbursts is grossly out of proportion to the provocation or to any precipitating psychosocial stressors.

C. The recurrent aggressive outbursts are not premeditated (i.e., they are impulsive and/or anger-based) and are not committed to achieve some tangible objective (e.g., money, power, intimidation).

D. The recurrent aggressive outbursts cause either marked distress in the individual or impairment in occupational or interpersonal functioning, or are associated with financial or legal consequences.

E. Chronological age is at least 6 years (or equivalent developmental level).

F. The recurrent aggressive outbursts are not better explained by another mental disorder (e.g., major depressive disorder, bipolar disorder, disruptive mood dysregulation disorder, a psychotic disorder, antisocial personality disorder, borderline personality disorder) and are not attributable to another medical condition (e.g., head trauma, Alzheimer's disease) or to the physiological effects of a substance (e.g., a drug of abuse, a medication). For children ages 6–18 years, aggressive behavior that occurs as part of an adjustment disorder should not be considered for this diagnosis.

Note: This diagnosis can be made in addition to the diagnosis of attention-deficit/hyperactivity disorder, conduct disorder, oppositional defiant disorder, or autism spectrum disorder when recurrent impulsive aggressive outbursts are in excess of those usually seen in these disorders and warrant independent clinical attention.

Gambling Disorder

A. Persistent and recurrent problematic gambling behavior leading to clinically significant impairment or distress, as indicated by the individual exhibiting four (or more) of the following in a 12-month period:

1. Needs to gamble with increasing amounts of money in order to achieve the desired excitement.
2. Is restless or irritable when attempting to cut down or stop gambling.
3. Has made repeated unsuccessful efforts to control, cut back, or stop gambling.
4. Is often preoccupied with gambling (e.g., having persistent thoughts of reliving past gambling experiences, handicapping or planning the next venture, thinking of ways to get money with which to gamble).
5. Often gambles when feeling distressed (e.g., helpless, guilty, anxious, depressed).
6. After losing money gambling, often returns another day to get even ("chasing" one's losses).
7. Lies to conceal the extent of involvement with gambling.
8. Has jeopardized or lost a significant relationship, job, or educational or career opportunity because of gambling.
9. Relies on others to provide money to relieve desperate financial situations caused by gambling.

B. The gambling behavior is not better explained by a manic episode.

Training Materials

Two types of sample cases are included for training: role-play cases and homework cases.

Role-Play Cases

Five role-play cases are useful for practicing how to administer the SCID-5-CV. These role-play cases work best in groups of two to four, with one person taking on the role of the SCID interviewer, a second person taking on the role of the patient, and the remaining participants acting as observers, making ratings along with the interviewer. Each case should be read by the "patient" only; the other members of the group should remain in the dark so that the psychopathology can be revealed as the role-play develops. The "patient" should start by reading the case Overview section aloud to the other members of the group. This is in lieu of doing the entire SCID-5-CV Overview, which we have found to be particularly difficult to role-play. The interviewer should then begin the practice interview with Module A. The person playing the patient should follow the instructions about how to answer the questions so that multiple small groups involved in the role-play case will arrive at the same diagnosis. After each role-play case, it is suggested that the entire group discuss the case together, focusing on any discrepancies within and between groups.

Homework Cases

Nine homework cases (adapted from the DSM-IV-TR Casebook [Spitzer et al. 2002], with some changes to facilitate the application of the diagnostic criteria) are intended to help the clinician practice how to navigate through Module C of the SCID-5-CV. When administering the SCID-5-CV, the clinician is expected to go through Modules C and D with the patient sitting in front of him or her, so the clinician has the opportunity to ask additional clarifying questions. It is therefore advisable for the clinician to become proficient in using Modules C and D before interviewing an actual patient. Each case should be read and then items rated as if administering the SCID-5-CV to that patient, starting at the beginning of Module A. If information for rating a particular criterion is not mentioned in the case vignette, assume it has not been present and assign a rating of "—." The discussion following each case indicates the correct "pathway" through the SCID-5-CV, providing the ratings for pertinent item labels in each case.

Role-Play Cases

Role-Play Case 1 (for practicing Modules A and B): "Depressed Truck Driver"

(Read this aloud to the interviewer)
Overview

This is a 50-year-old divorced male who reports having been depressed for the past 6 months. He works as a truck driver but is in danger of losing his job from missing so much work lately. He reports that some days he'll just sit on the edge of his bed, staring at the floor, unable to move. He also reports that he has been avoiding his friends and no longer·likes to venture out of the house. He had a similar episode 10 years ago when he was going through a divorce. Between these episodes he has felt well.

(For the role-play)

Mood symptoms: For the period of the current month (no 2-week period has been particularly worse than the others), report depressive symptoms as follows:

- Acknowledge persistent depression (Criterion A1).
- Acknowledge loss of interest (Criterion A2).
- Acknowledge loss of appetite accompanied by a 20-pound weight loss (Criterion A3).
- Acknowledge trouble falling asleep (tossing and turning for 2 hours) and then waking up at 5 A.M. (Criterion A4).
- Deny psychomotor agitation (first part of Criterion A5) but acknowledge severe psychomotor retardation (Criterion A5). (Alternatively, you can demonstrate the severe psychomotor retardation if your acting skills are up to it.)
- Acknowledge fatigue or loss of energy (Criterion A6).
- Deny feelings of worthlessness and report feelings of guilt (Criterion A7), but do not give details unless the interviewer asks for them. When asked about guilt, say that you are feeling very guilty and provide an example that is clearly excessive (e.g., explain that your son has a serious drug problem, and you are convinced that it's because you were on the road so much and didn't spend time playing with him when he was a little boy).
- Deny difficulty concentrating or making decisions (Criterion A8).
- Deny suicidal ideation (Criterion A9).

If the interviewer asks about how the depression has affected your life, remind the interviewer that you have been unable to work because of the depression and that although you have lived alone since your divorce 10 years ago, you have a lot of good friends. However, because of your depression, you have isolated yourself from them. You are in good health and have not started using (nor increased the amount of) alcohol, drugs, or medications. When asked how many separate times in your life that you have been depressed, say two times—now and 10 years ago.

The next question to you should be about whether you have been manic in the last month. Answer "NO" to the question about whether there was a period of time in the past month when you were feeling good, high, or excited. Answer "YES" to the question about whether during the current month you had a period when you were irritable, angry, or short-tempered most of the day. Explain that when you get depressed, you get very irritable and short-tempered and any little thing can set you off. Answer "NO," however, to the follow-up question about feeling "hyper" and having an unusual amount of energy. As you explained earlier, you feel slowed down and have no energy at all. The interviewer should (hopefully) skip to the question about past Manic Episode. Deny that there have ever been any past episodes of elevated or irritable mood. Also deny feeling down for more days than not in the past 2 years.

Psychotic and associated symptoms: Answer "NO" to everything except the following:

1. Answer "YES" to the first question about whether people pay special attention to you. Explain that you stay inside because if you go out, you run into people who keep asking why you're not at work.
2. Answer "YES" to the second question about delusions of guilt ("Have you ever felt that something you did, or should have done but did not do, caused serious harm to your parents, children, other family members, or friends?"). Reiterate how terribly guilty you feel that you are the cause of your son's drug addiction because you did not play with him enough when he was a little boy because you were away so much. You do understand that you feel this way because you are depressed and that these feelings are probably exaggerated because of this.

SCID-5-CV diagnosis

F33.2   Major Depressive Disorder, Recurrent, Severe
("Current" box checked on Diagnostic Summary Score Sheet)

Role-Play Case 2 (for practicing Modules A and B): "World Peace Through Meditation"

(Read this aloud to the interviewer)
Overview

This divorced 30-year-old woman is brought to the hospital by her family, because over the past 3 weeks she has quit her job as a receptionist in a doctor's office, put her house on the market, and has not been sleeping; her behavior has been increasingly bizarre. She is very angry about her hospitalization, believing that her family just wants to prevent her from sharing her good news with the world.

(For the role-play)

Mood symptoms: Answer "never" to all questions about depression and loss of interest. In response to the question about feeling good, "high," excited, or "on top of the world," explain that you are feeling "joyous" about quitting your old job and your newly discovered ability to teach meditation, and that you have been feeling this way for over 3 weeks now. In response to the follow-up question about being "hyper" or "wired," explain that you also have a tremendous amount of energy to do things and that you are thrilled about all of the great things that you have been doing and are about to do.

For the Criterion B symptoms:

- When asked about how you feel about yourself (Criterion B1), say that you feel great, that you are especially excited about discovering that you have a special power to teach other people how to meditate "through osmosis," and that you are going to bring about world peace by opening a meditation center in California. When the interviewer (hopefully) asks you for more details about how this works, explain that you can teach people to meditate simply by staring at them intently for a few minutes and then they can meditate. You know you have been successful because of the look in their eyes after you do it.
- When asked about your sleeping (Criterion B2), say that you have not slept for 10 days because you are so excited about your new powers.
- When asked about talking too much (Criterion B3), either demonstrate overtalkativeness or tell the interviewer that your family is complaining that you talk too much.
- When asked about racing thoughts (Criterion B4), say your mind is "flooded" with ideas about your new meditation center.
- When asked about distractibility (Criterion B5), say "YES," but you are unable to give any examples.
- When asked about increase in activities (Criterion B6), say you have been going all over town to TV and radio stations trying to get the news out.
- When asked about doing anything that could get you in trouble (Criterion B7), say that you got arrested when you tried to barge into the NBC Nightly News studios to share your message on air.

You are now and always have been in excellent health and you deny having taken any alcohol or drugs of any kind for the past several years.

Psychotic symptoms: Answer "NO" to the question regarding people talking about you or taking special notice of you. In response to being asked about receiving special messages from the TV, explain that it's your message you've been trying to get to the TV people. Answer "NO" to the questions about having the feeling that the words in a song, what people were wearing, or street signs or billboards were meant to give you a message.

About persecutory delusions, say your family thinks you're crazy because they fail to understand the importance of your new powers, and you're very angry with them for railroading you into the hospital. Answer "NO" to the question about having the feeling of being followed or spied on and "NO" to the question about being poisoned.

In response to questions about having special powers, respond by saying "How did you find out? Is it all over the news already?" and explain again about your power to teach people to meditate through osmosis, and how once everyone can do this, there will no longer be any need for war and that is why there will be world peace. Answer "NO" to the question about having a close relationship with someone famous.

Answer "NO" to the questions about being convinced that something is wrong with you physically or that something strange is happening to parts of your body. Answer "NO" to the questions about having committed a crime or that you have done something that has caused serious harm to the family.

Answer "NO" to the question about being convinced that a partner was unfaithful. Answer "YES" to the question about whether you are a religious or spiritual person, explaining that you were raised Catholic and used to go to church every Sunday, but although you no longer go regularly you still consider yourself religious. Then answer "NO" to the question about having any religious or spiritual experiences that other people have not experienced and "NO" to the question about whether God, the devil, or some other spiritual being has communicated directly with you.

Answer "NO" to the question about a secret admirer or being involved romantically with someone famous. Answer "NO" to the remaining delusional questions about feeling controlled, having thoughts put into your head, having thoughts taken out of your head, feeling that your thoughts were being broadcast out loud, or believing that someone can read your mind.

In response to the question about hearing voices, say that sometimes you hear your name being called. When that happens, you turn in the direction from where you've heard it, but no one is there. Say "NO" to all other hallucinations.

SCID-5-CV diagnosis

F31.2   Bipolar I Disorder, Current Episode Manic, With Psychotic Features
("Current" box checked on Diagnostic Summary Score Sheet)

Role-Play Case 3 (for practicing Modules A, B, and C): "The Stalker"

(Read this aloud to the interviewer)

Overview

This is a single 35-year-old female administrative assistant who says she has been "pursued" by a police officer ever since she appeared in court for a speeding ticket 10 months ago.

(For the role-play)

Mood symptoms: In response to questions about current depression, say your mood is "distraught" and "upset" and that you've felt that way for weeks, but answer "NO" to feeling sad, depressed, down, or hopeless. Answer "NO" to the question about whether you have lost interest or pleasure in things you enjoyed. If the interviewer decides to continue with the questions for a current depressive episode, answer "NO" to all of the depressive symptom questions except answer "YES" to the question about having trouble falling asleep (Criterion A4) and "YES" to the question about having trouble concentrating (Criterion A8), because you are so frightened about what the police officer means to do to you.

Answer "NO" to the question about having had any other times in the past when you have felt depressed or down and "NO" to the question about ever having lost interest or pleasure in things you usually enjoyed.

Answer "NO" to current and past manic questions (i.e., you never had any periods of feeling so good, "high," excited, or "on top of the world" that other people thought you were not your normal self and never had any periods of feeling irritable, angry, or short-tempered lasting for at least several days).

In response to the initial question for current Persistent Depressive Disorder (item label A78; "Since (TWO YEARS AGO), have you been bothered by depressed mood most of the day, more days than not?"), say that while the court appearance occurred 10 months ago, it's only in the last few weeks that you've realized he is stalking you and have been so upset. If asked, clarify that therefore, you have not been depressed more days than not in the past 2 years.

Psychotic symptoms: In response to the initial question about whether people were talking about you or taking special notice of you, explain that the police officer is the only one who has taken special notice of you. You know this because you see him hanging around outside your building at night. And you get hang-ups on your telephone that you're sure are from him. Deny the other questions about delusions of reference (i.e., deny that things on the radio, TV, newspaper, songs, what people are wearing, and street signs or billboards have any special meaning for you).

In response to the question about whether someone is going out of their way to give you a hard time or try to hurt you, say you're not sure why the policeman is doing this or what he wants from you, but you think it's something sexual. Answer "YES" to the question that you have the feeling that you are being followed by the policeman but that you don't know why. If asked, you should explain that you are absolutely sure that he is following you and that is it not just your imagination.

Answer "NO" to the question about being especially important or having special powers and "NO" to the question about having a close relationship with someone famous.

Answer "NO" to the questions about being convinced that something is wrong with you physically or that something strange is happening to parts of your body. Answer "NO" to the questions about committing a crime or that you had done something that caused serious harm to your family.

Answer "NO" to the question about being convinced that a partner was unfaithful. Answer "NO" to the question about whether you are a religious or spiritual person, and then "NO" again to the question about feeling that God, the devil, or some other spiritual being or higher power has communicated directly with you.

Answer "NO" to the question about a secret admirer or being involved romantically with someone famous. Answer "NO" to the remaining delusional questions about feeling controlled, having thoughts put into your head, having thoughts taken out of your head, feeling that your thoughts were being broadcast out loud, or believing that someone could read your mind. Answer "NO" to all of the other questions about delusions.

Answer "NO" to all of the questions about hallucinations. If the interviewer inquires further about visual hallucinations (given that you have said that you have "seen" him hanging around building), explain that you have seen what looks to you like this police officer night after night, driving up and down the street, pretending to patrol the neighborhood—and that although he is not close enough for you to actually see his features, you are sure it is him.

If asked, deny that there has been a recent period of time when you were not working, not in school, or unable to take care of things.

You have no medical problems and deny any drug or alcohol use, and you are not taking any medications.

SCID-5-CV diagnosis

F22 **Delusional Disorder**
(*"Current" box checked on Diagnostic Summary Score Sheet*)

Role-Play Case 4 (for practicing Modules F and G): "Better Safe Than Sorry"

(Read this aloud to the interviewer)
Overview

This 28-year-old, married Latina mother of two small children is seeking treatment for panic attacks and worry that have become progressively more disturbing to her. She describes having panic attacks that started about 2 years ago and have become more frequent over the past year. For the past year, she has also been avoiding any setting where there might be a crowd because she's worried about being trapped if she might have a panic attack and be unable to escape, such as in crowded, small shops. Even if the shop were not to be crowded, because it could become crowded at a moment's notice she will avoid it, explaining that it's better to be safe than sorry.

(For the role-play)

Mood symptoms: Answer "NO" to all the questions about mood symptoms: you've never been depressed for more than a day or two at a time, have never been abnormally elated or irritable, and have not been depressed more days than not in the last 2 years.

Psychotic symptoms: Answer "NO" to everything.

Substance use disorders: You may occasionally drink a glass of wine with dinner when you go out, but alcohol never caused any problems. You tried marijuana once in college, but it just made you sleepy.

Anxiety symptoms: Answer "YES" to the initial panic attack question and describe the last bad one you had, which was yesterday. You were sitting at home watching TV, and it suddenly came out of nowhere. When you describe it, tell the interviewer how your heart was racing, you were sweating, you felt faint, and you were short of breath. Acknowledge that the symptoms came on all of a sudden and got bad within a few minutes.

In response to the questions about specific symptoms associated with the panic attack:

- Answer "YES" to the question about your heart racing (Criterion A1).
- Answer "YES" to sweating (Criterion A2).
- Answer "YES" to trembling (Criterion A3).
- Answer "YES" to shortness of breath (Criterion A4).
- Answer "NO" to feelings of choking (Criterion A5).
- Answer "YES" to chest pain (Criterion A6).
- Answer "NO" to nausea or abdominal distress (Criterion A7).
- Answer "YES" to feeling dizzy (Criterion A8).
- Answer "NO" to flushes or hot flashes (Criterion A9).
- Answer "YES" to tingling (say it was in your hands) (Criterion A10).
- Answer "NO" to derealization (Criterion A11).

- Answer "NO" to fear of losing control (Criterion A12).
- Answer "NO" to fear of dying (Criterion A13).

When the interviewer asks if any of these attacks came on out of the blue, say that most of the panic attacks seem to come on without anything going on that might be making you anxious, like the attack that happened while you were watching TV. When the interviewer asks whether you have been concerned or worried that you might have another attack, answer "YES." You are always worried about having another attack—you constantly think about it, wondering when the next one is going to happen. When the interviewer asks whether you have done anything differently because of the attacks, tell the interviewer that you avoid any situation in which you might be stuck in a crowd of people...situations like a crowded store, a crowded bus, a crowded movie theatre, even a crowded elevator. You are constantly scoping out your environment; if you see that a bus, a store, or an elevator is too crowded or looks like it might become crowded, you simply will not go in. This has been going on for the past year.

In response to the question about when the panic attacks started, say that they first started about 2 years ago but that they have been getting more frequent recently. You were not taking any medication or using any drugs when they started, and you always only drink decaffeinated coffee and herbal teas because caffeine has always made you jumpy. You were not physically ill when the panic attacks started. In fact, after the first panic attack you went to the doctor because you thought something was wrong with your heart, but the doctor gave you a clean bill of health.

When asked about the past month, say that you have had panic attacks daily. In response to the question about being concerned about having attacks in the past month, say that you have constantly been worried about having more panic attacks. Finally, in response to the question about doing anything different, reiterate that you avoid crowded places.

Answer "YES" to the question about being anxious about or afraid of a number of situations in the past 6 months (Criterion A) and describe briefly again the situations that you avoid (i.e., any situation that might be crowded). You avoid crowded buses, but if the bus is not crowded, you will take it. You do not avoid traveling on any other form of transportation. You do not avoid open spaces like parking lots, outdoor marketplaces, or bridges because they generally do not get crowded. You usually avoid enclosed places like stores, movie theaters, and shopping malls because even if they are not crowded, at any time they might be, so it's better to be safe than sorry. You do not avoid being out of the house alone.

When asked about what you are afraid would happen, explain that you are afraid of having a panic attack and that the crowd would make it hard for you to get out (Criterion B). Since about a year ago, you always feel anxious or frightened in crowded situations (Criterion C), and you go out of your way to avoid such situations (Criterion D). Although you are afraid that you will not be able to escape, there is nothing especially dangerous or threatening to you about crowds (Criterion E). This fear has been present for most of the past year (Criterion F). When asked about the effect on your life, say that this anxiety and fear make it very difficult to take care of your family because of all the places you avoid. You will not go into any small stores because they might become crowded, and you will not go into any large stores or shopping malls during times of the day when they might be crowded, such as on weekends. You are very bothered by the fact that you have these fears.

Answer "NO" to the question about being especially nervous in social situations but answer "YES" to the question about whether in the past 6 months you have been afraid to do things in front of other people (Criterion A). Explain, however, that this is limited to being nervous about speaking in front of large groups of people and that you think this is not any more than most people would feel. Deny that there are any other social or performance situations that make your nervous (Criterion A).

If the interviewer chooses to continue with the Social Anxiety Disorder assessment:

- To the question "What were you afraid would happen when you had to speak in front of a large group of people?" explain that you would be afraid of being embarrassed by saying something stupid (Criterion B).
- Answer "YES" to the question "Have you almost always felt frightened when you have to speak in front of a large group of people?" (Criterion C).
- In response to the question "Have you gone out of your way to avoid speaking in front of people?" answer that in those few instances where you had to speak in front of a group of other people, like in class in high school, you would skip class (Criterion D).
- When asked what would be the likely outcome of a bad performance speaking in front of a large group, say that you would be embarrassed but nothing else would happen (Criterion E).
- When asked about whether your fear or avoidance has been present for most of the past 6 months, say that you have felt this way since you were a child (Criterion F).
- When asked what effect this fear of speaking in front of large groups has had on your life, say that it has had very little impact because such situations rarely arise and there are no negative implications for avoiding speaking in front of large groups of people (Criterion G).

Answer "YES" to the question about whether you have felt anxious and worried for a lot of the time over the last 6 months. Explain that in addition to your fears about having a panic attack, you find yourself racked with worry about almost everything. You worry about whether your husband will get killed while on a business trip, about whether your children will develop a deadly illness, about your finances (despite the fact that your husband assures you that he is making a good living and his job is secure), about whether you are being a good enough mother, and so forth. Acknowledge that you worry even when there is no reason and that your husband is constantly saying that you worry too much. Answer "YES" to the question about whether you have been worrying more days than not over the past 6 months.

In response to the question "When you're worrying this way, have you found that it's hard to stop yourself or to think about anything else?" answer that you often tell yourself it's ridiculous to be worrying, but your mind keeps drifting back to whatever you've been worrying about.

In response to the Generalized Anxiety Disorder symptom questions:

- Answer "YES" to feeling on edge (Criterion C1).
- Answer "YES" to feeling tired a lot of the time (Criterion C2).
- Answer "NO" to having trouble concentrating (Criterion C3).
- Answer "NO" to irritability (Criterion C4).
- Answer "NO" to muscle tension (Criterion C5).
- Answer "YES" to having trouble getting to sleep because you think about all the things that might go wrong (Criterion C6).

In response to what effect this has had on your life, answer that you need to call your husband every day to make sure that he can pick up the kids after work and he finds this very annoying; this is causing a lot of strain on your relationship with him. You are also very critical of yourself for being this way and wish you could loosen up.

You do not have any medical problems, you do not drink or use drugs, and you do not drink more than one cup of coffee a day.

Answer "NO" to the three screening questions about obsessions (i.e., thoughts that kept coming back, images that kept coming back, and urges that kept coming back). Answer "YES" to the question about whether there was something you had to do over and over again. Explain that you have to go back in the house almost every time you leave to check that the stove is off, the iron turned off, the electric heater unplugged, and so forth. This behavior is ritualized in that it must be done in a certain order or else you have to start all over again. This checking behavior ends up taking only about 5–10 minutes a day, and you insist that you are NOT bothered by it and that it does NOT significantly interfere with your life.

SCID-5-CV diagnoses

F41.0　　**Panic Disorder**
F40.00　**Agoraphobia**
F41.1　　**Generalized Anxiety Disorder**
(*"Current" box checked on Diagnostic Summary Score Sheet for all three diagnoses*)

Role-Play Case 5 (for practicing Module E): "Too Busy"

(Read this aloud to the interviewer)

Overview

This 40-year-old Mexican American male has been admitted to a drug treatment program. He has never been married and lives alone. He is a swimming pool contractor currently in the midst of his busy season, working 60 hours a week, and spending evenings at the hospital visiting his terminally ill mother. He reports that the main drug he uses is cocaine and that "it's gotten out of control." He has been spending more than $300 a week on it. As far as his drinking habits go, he reports drinking two glasses of wine with dinner and an additional two to three beers when he goes out with friends in the evening, which is about two times a week.

(For the role-play)

Mood symptoms: Answer "YES" to the current depressed mood question, but when the interviewer asks about whether the depressed mood is present "most of the day, nearly every day," say "NO." You are depressed about your mother, but you don't think about it during the day because you're so busy. In response to loss of interest, say again that you don't have time to do anything but work, visit your mother, and sleep— but you are still interested in work and visiting your mother. If the interviewer (incorrectly) asks the current depressive episode questions, answer "NO" to all of them. Answer "NO" to all other questions in the mood module.

Psychotic symptoms: Answer "NO" to everything, except for vivid, brightly colored "auras" (visual illusions—NOT hallucinations) when you were high on LSD.

Substance use disorders: As you described in the Overview, you have been drinking two glasses of wine with dinner and, a couple of nights a week, you have an additional two to three beers when you go out with your friends. With regard to the questions evaluating Alcohol Use Disorder in the past 12 months, say "NO" to all 11 of the Alcohol Use Disorder questions: the drinking has not caused any problems in the past 12 months nor is it out of control.

When asked about nonalcohol substance use in the past 12 months, answer the questions as follows:

- Deny using any drugs from the Sedatives, Hypnotics, or Anxiolytics class.
- Acknowledge smoking marijuana every day, three or four joints, sometimes beginning right after breakfast.
- Acknowledge snorting cocaine daily. Deny using any other kinds of stimulants.
- Deny using any opioids.
- Deny using any PCP.
- Acknowledge using LSD about once a month during the past year.
- Deny using any inhalants.
- Deny using any other types of drugs.

For the assessment of the criteria for Past-12-Month Nonalcohol Substance Use Disorder, the interviewer should ask you which drugs or medications caused you the most problems over the past 12 months. You should say "definitely the cocaine." Then answer the individual questions as follows:

Criterion A1 (taking more than intended)
Answer "YES"—Your cocaine use is out of control; you often use up all your cocaine in one evening, even when you had an amount that should last for a week.

Criterion A2 (persistent desire or unsuccessful efforts to cut down)
Answer "YES"—You have tried to stop many times, but have not been able to stop—that is why you have come for treatment.

Criterion A3 (great deal of time spent)
Answer "YES"—You have been using it every day, and you're "coked up" all the time while working on the swimming pools.

Criterion A4 (craving)
Answer "YES"—You always crave it when you are not using it.

Criterion A5 (use resulting in failure to fulfill major role obligations)
Answer "NO"—Although you might be a bit speedy at work, you have been if anything more productive; there has not been any negative impact on role obligations.

Criterion A6 (continued use despite having social problems)
Answer "YES"—Your family disapproves of your drug use; every time you speak with them, it turns into an argument about your cocaine use. Recently you have avoided speaking with anyone in your family because you don't want to be hassled anymore.

Criterion A7 (activities given up)
Answer "YES"—You have stopped spending time with family and friends, and you no longer play sports, which is something that was once your main interest.

Criterion A8 (use when physically hazardous)
Answer "YES" to the question about whether you have snorted cocaine before driving but answer "NO" to the question about your cocaine use causing reckless or risky driving.

Criterion A9 (use despite knowledge of psychological or physical problem)
Answer "YES" to psychological problems—Earlier in the year, when you were using even higher doses of cocaine, it would make you very paranoid; you would lock the doors of your house and become convinced that the police were watching you.
Answer "NO" to physical problems.
Answer "YES" to whether you kept using cocaine anyway.

Criterion A10 (tolerance)
Answer "YES"—You needed to escalate the amount used after only a few days.

Criterion A11 (withdrawal)
Answer "YES"—After you run out of cocaine, you "crash" and become depressed and irritable, sleep all the time, feel fatigued, and be slowed down.

SCID-5-CV diagnosis

F14.20   Cocaine Use Disorder, Severe
(Criteria A1, A2, A3, A4, A6, A7, A8, A9, A10, A11)
(*"Current" box checked on Diagnostic Summary Score Sheet*)

Homework Cases

Homework Case 1: "Low Life Level"

Ms. Larkin, age 39 years, is a pale, stooped, single white woman. Her childlike face is surrounded by scraggly blond braids tied with pink ribbons. She was referred for a psychiatric evaluation for possible hospitalization by her family doctor who was concerned about her low level of functioning. Her only complaint to him was: "I have a decline in self-care and a low life level." Her mother reports that there has indeed been a decline, but that it has been over many years. In the last few months she has remained in her room, mute and still.

Twelve years ago Ms. Larkin was a supervisor in the occupational therapy department of a large hospital, lived in her own apartment, and was engaged to a young man. He broke the engagement, and she became increasingly disorganized, wandering aimlessly in the street, wearing mismatched clothing. She was fired from her job, and eventually the police were called to hospitalize her. They broke into her apartment, which was in shambles, filled with papers, food, and broken objects. No information is available from this hospitalization, which lasted 3 months, and from which she was discharged to her mother's house with a prescription for unknown medication that she never filled.

After her discharge her family hoped that she would gather herself together and embark again on a real life, but as the years progressed she became more withdrawn and less functional. Most of her time was spent watching TV and cooking. Her cooking consisted of mixing bizarre combinations of ingredients, such as broccoli and cake mix, and she ate alone because no one else in the family would eat her meals. She collected cookbooks and recipes, cluttering her room with stacks of these. Often when her mother entered her room, she would quickly grab a magazine and pretend to be reading, when in fact she had apparently just been sitting and staring into space. She stopped bathing and brushing her hair or teeth. She ate less and less, although she denied loss of appetite, and over a period of several years lost 20 pounds. She would sleep at odd hours. Eventually she became enuretic, wetting her bed frequently and filling the room with the pungent odor of urine.

On admission to the psychiatric hospital, she sat with her hands tightly clasped in her lap and avoided looking at the doctor who interviewed her. She answered questions readily and did not appear suspicious or guarded, but her affect was shallow. She denied depressed mood, delusions, or hallucinations; however, her answers became increasingly idiosyncratic and irrelevant as the interview progressed. In response to a question about her strange cooking habits, she replied that she did not wish to discuss recent events in Russia. When discussing her decline in functioning, she said, "There's more of a take-off mechanism when you're younger." Asked about ideas of reference, she said, "I doubt it's true, but if one knows the writers involved, it could be an element that would be directed in a comical way." Her answers were interspersed with the mantra, "I'm safe. I'm safe."

SCID-5-CV Rating for "Low Life Level"

Module A	Item Label, Rating, and Notes
Page 10:	A1 = "—"; A2 = "—"
Page 13:	A15 = "—"; A16 = "—"
Page 17:	A29 = "—"
Page 22:	A54 = "—"
Page 29:	A78 = "—"

Module B	Item Label, Rating, and Notes
Page 31:	B1–B2 = "—"
Page 32:	B3–B7 = "—"
Page 33:	B8–B14 = "—"
Page 34:	B15–B19 = "—"

Page 34: B20 = + (*disorganized speech*: "answers became increasingly idiosyncratic and irrelevant"; "I doubt it's true, but if one knows the writers involved, it could be an element that would be directed in a comical way")

Page 35: B21 = + (*grossly disorganized behavior*: "she became increasingly disorganized, wandering aimlessly in the street, wearing mismatched clothing")

B22 = "—"

Page 36: B23 = "+" (*avolition*: "sitting and staring into space"; "stopped bathing and brushing her hair or teeth")

B24 = "+" (*diminished emotional expressiveness*: "her affect was shallow")

Module C	Item Label, Rating, and Notes
Page 37:	C1 = "YES" (psychotic symptoms outside of mood episodes)

C2 = "YES" (disorganized speech, disorganized behavior, and negative symptoms occurring together for at least a month)

C3 = "YES" (no mood episode ever)

Page 38: C4 = "YES" (continuous signs of illness for years)

C5 = "YES" (severe functional impairment)

C6 = "YES" (not due to a GMC or substance/medication)

Page 44: C25 = "+" (symptoms present at some point during past month)

On the Diagnostic Summary Score Sheet, the "Current" box preceding F20.9 Schizophrenia should be checked.

SCID-5-CV diagnosis: Schizophrenia

Homework Case 2: "I Am Vishnu"

Mr. Nehru is a 32-year-old single, unemployed man who migrated from India to the United States when he was 13. His brother brought him to the emergency room of an Atlanta, Georgia, hospital after neighbors complained that he was standing in the street harassing people about his religious beliefs. To the psychiatrist he keeps repeating, "I am Vishnu. I am Krishna."

Mr. Nehru has been living with his brother and sister-in-law for the past 7 months. During the last 4 weeks, his behavior has become increasingly disruptive. He awakens his brother at all hours of the night to discuss religious matters. He often seems to be responding to voices that only he hears. He neither bathes nor changes his clothes.

Mr. Nehru states that about 6 weeks ago, he started hearing "voices." There are several voices, which comment on his behavior and discuss him in the third person. They usually are either benign (e.g., "Look at him now. He is about to eat") or insulting in content (e.g., "What a fool he is—he doesn't understand anything!"). During this time he watches little TV, because he hears the voices coming out of the TV and is upset that the TV shows often refer to him.

For the past 6 weeks, with increasing insistence, the voices have been telling Mr. Nehru that he is the new Messiah, Jesus, Moses, Vishnu, and Krishna and should begin a new religious epoch in human history. Starting about 4 weeks ago, he began to experience surges of increased energy, "so I could spread my gospel," and needs very little sleep. According to his brother, he has become more preoccupied with the voices and disorganized in his daily activities.

When interviewed, Mr. Nehru is euphoric, and his speech is rapid and hard to follow. He paces up and down the ward and, upon seeing a doctor, grabs his arm, puts his face within 2 inches of the doctor's, and talks with great rapidity and enthusiasm about his religious "insights." In the middle of a speech on his new religion, he abruptly compliments the doctor on how well his shirt and tie match. When limits are placed on his behavior, he becomes loud and angry. In addition to his belief that he is the Messiah, he feels that the hospital is part of a conspiracy to suppress his religious message. He is troubled by the voices that he hears throughout the day, sometimes referring to them as "those damned voices." He states that he feels that his religious insights, euphoria, and energy have been put into him by God.

SCID-5-CV Rating for "I Am Vishnu"

Module A	Item Label, Rating, and Notes
Page 10:	A1 = "—"; A2 = "—"
Page 13:	A15 = "—"; A16 = "—"
Page 17:	A29 = "—"
Page 22:	A54 = "—"
Page 29:	A78 = "—"

Module B	Item Label, Rating, and Notes
Page 31:	B1 = "+" ("the TV shows often refer to him")
Page 31:	B2 = "+" ("the hospital is part of a conspiracy to suppress his religious message")
Page 32:	B3 = "+" ("he is the new Messiah")
	B4–B6 = "—"
	B7 = "+" ("he is the new Messiah")
Page 33:	B8–B13 = "—"
	B14 = "+" ("several voices...comment on his behavior and discuss him in the third person"; "voices have been telling Mr. Nehru that he is the new Messiah, Jesus, Moses, Vishnu, and Krishna"; "He is troubled by voices that he hears throughout the day")
Page 34:	B15–B20 = "—"
Page 35:	B21–B22 = "—"
Page 36:	B23–B24 = "—"

Module C	Item Label, Rating, and Notes
Page 37:	C1 = "YES" (psychotic symptoms outside of mood episodes)
	C2 = "YES" (delusions and hallucinations)
	C3 = "NO" (there ARE Manic Episodes concurrent with active-phase symptoms of Schizophrenia and the mood episodes are NOT present for only a minority of the time [i.e., they are present for a majority of the time])
Page 39:	C9 = "YES" (manic symptoms concurrent with active symptoms of Schizophrenia)
	C10 = "YES" (auditory hallucinations in the absence of prominent mood symptoms)
Page 40:	C11 = "YES" (mood episode symptoms for a majority of the time)
	C12 = "YES" (not due to a GMC or substance/medication)
Page 44:	C27 = "+" (symptoms present at some point during past month)
	On the Diagnostic Summary Score Sheet, the "Current" box preceding F25.0 Schizoaffective Disorder, Bipolar Type, should be checked.

SCID-5-CV diagnosis:　Schizoaffective Disorder, Bipolar Type

Homework Case 3: "Contract on My Life"

Mr. Polsen, a 42-year-old married, African American postal worker and father of two, is brought to the emergency room by his wife because he has been insisting that "there is a contract out on my life."

According to Mr. Polsen, his problems began 4 months ago when his supervisor at work accused him of tampering with a package. Mr. Polsen denied that this was true and, because his job was in jeopardy, filed a protest. At a formal hearing, he was exonerated and, according to him, "This made my boss furious. He felt he had been publicly humiliated."

About 2 weeks later, Mr. Polsen noticed that his coworkers were avoiding him. "When I'd walk toward them, they'd just turn away like they didn't want to see me." Shortly thereafter, he began to feel that they were talking about him at work. He never could make out clearly what they were saying, but he gradually became convinced that they were avoiding him because his boss had taken out a contract on his life.

This state of affairs was stable for about 2 months, until Mr. Polsen began noticing several "large white cars," new to his neighborhood, driving up and down the street on which he lived. He became increasingly frightened and was convinced that the "hit men" were in these cars. He refused to go out of his apartment without an escort. Several times, when he saw the white cars, he would panic and run home. After the latest such incident, his wife finally insisted that he accompany her to the emergency room.

Mr. Polsen was described by his wife and brother as a basically well-adjusted, outgoing man who enjoyed being with his family. He had served with distinction in Iraq. He saw little combat there, but was pulled from a burning truck by a buddy seconds before the truck blew up.

When interviewed, Mr. Polsen was obviously frightened. Aside from his belief that he was in danger of being killed, his speech, behavior, and demeanor were in no way odd or strange. His predominant mood was anxious. He denied having hallucinations and all other psychotic symptoms except those noted above. He claimed not to be depressed, and although he noted that he had recently had some difficulty falling asleep, he said there had been no change in his appetite, sex drive, energy level, or concentration.

SCID-5-CV Rating for "Contract on My Life"

Module A   **Item Label, Rating, and Notes**

Page 10:   A1 = "—"; A2 = "—"

Page 13:   A15 = "—"; A16 = "—"

Page 17:   A29 = "—"

Page 22:   A54 = "—"

Page 29:   A78 = "—"

Module B   **Item Label, Rating, and Notes**

Page 31:   B1 = "+" ("hit men" in white cars; coworkers turning away)

                B2 = "+" (boss put out a contract on his life)

Page 32:   B3–B7 = "—"

Page 33:   B8–B14 = "—"

Page 34:   B15–B20 = "—"

Page 35:   B21–B22 = "—"

Page 36:   B23–B24 = "—"

Module C   **Item Label, Rating, and Notes**

Page 37:   C1 = "YES" (no mood episodes ever)

                C2 = "NO" (delusions only)

Page 40:   C13 = "YES" (delusions for more than 1 month)

                C14 = "YES" (no history of Schizophrenia)

                C15 = "YES" (functioning is not markedly impaired and behavior is not
                obviously odd or bizarre)

Page 41:   C16 = "YES" (no mood episodes)

                C17 = "YES" (not due to a GMC or substance/medication)

                C18 = "YES" (not explained by another mental disorder)

Page 44:   C28 = "+" (symptoms present at some point during past month)

                On the Diagnostic Summary Score Sheet, the "Current" box preceding
                F22 Delusional Disorder should be checked.

SCID-5-CV diagnosis: Delusional Disorder

Homework Case 4: "The Socialite"

Ms. Cabot, a 42-year-old married white socialite, has never had any mental problems before. A new performance hall is to be formally opened with the world premiere of a new ballet, and Ms. Cabot, because of her position on the cultural council, has assumed the responsibility for coordinating that event. However, construction problems, including strikes, have made it uncertain whether finishing details will meet the deadline. The set designer has been volatile, threatening to walk out on the project unless the materials meet his meticulous specifications. Ms. Cabot has had to calm this volatile man while attempting to coax disputing groups to negotiate. She has also had increased responsibilities at home since her housekeeper had to leave to visit a sick relative.

In the midst of these difficulties, her best friend was decapitated in a tragic auto crash. Ms. Cabot is an only child, and her best friend had been very close to her since grade school. People often commented that the two women were like sisters.

Immediately following the funeral, Ms. Cabot became increasingly tense and jittery, and could sleep only 2–3 hours a night. Two days later she happened to see a woman driving a car just like the one her friend had driven. She was puzzled, and after a few hours she became convinced that her friend was alive and that the accident had been staged, along with the funeral, as part of a plot. Somehow the plot is directed toward deceiving her, and she senses that somehow she is in great danger and must solve the mystery to escape alive. She begins to distrust everyone except her husband, and begins to believe that the phone is tapped and that the rooms are "bugged." She pleads with her husband to help save her life. She begins to hear a high-pitched, undulating sound, which she fears is an ultrasound beam aimed at her. She is in a state of sheer panic, gripping her husband's arm in terror, as he brings her to the emergency room the next morning.

SCID-5-CV Rating for "The Socialite"

Module A	Item Label, Rating, and Notes
Page 10:	A1 = "—"; A2 = "—"
Page 13:	A15 = "—"; A16 = "—"
Page 17:	A29 = "—"
Page 22:	A54 = "—"
Page 29:	A78 = "—"

Module B	Item Label, Rating, and Notes
Page 31:	B1 = "+" (sees woman driving a car like the one her friend had driven—convinced this means her friend is alive)
	B2 = "+" (plot to deceive her; phone is tapped; room is bugged; she is in danger)
Page 32:	B3–B7 = "—"
Page 33:	B8–B13 = "—"
	B14 = "+" (high-pitched "ultrasound")
Page 34:	B15–B20 = "—"
Page 35:	B21–B22 = "—"
Page 36:	B23–B24 = "—"

Module C	Item Label, Rating, and Notes
Page 37:	C1 = "YES" (no mood episodes ever)
	C2 = "NO" (both delusions and hallucinations but lasted less than 1 month)
Page 40:	C13 = "NO" (delusions lasted less than 1 month)
Page 41:	C19 = "YES" (both delusions and hallucinations)
Page 42:	C20 = "YES" (delusions and hallucinations that lasted at least 1 day but less than 1 month)
	C21 = "YES" (not better explained by another mental disorder and not due to a GMC or substance/medication)
Page 44:	C29 = "+" (delusions and hallucinations present in the past month)
	On the Diagnostic Summary Score Sheet, the "Current" box preceding F23 Brief Psychotic Disorder should be checked.

SCID-5-CV diagnosis: Brief Psychotic Disorder

Homework Case 5: "Under Surveillance"

Mr. Simpson is a 44-year-old, single, unemployed white man brought into the emergency room by the police for striking an elderly woman in his apartment building. His chief complaint is, "That damn bitch. She and the rest of them deserved more than that for what they put me through."

He has been continuously ill since the age of 22. During his first year of law school, he gradually became more and more convinced that his classmates were making fun of him. He noticed that they would snort and sneeze whenever he entered the classroom. When a girl he was dating broke off the relationship with him, he believed that she had been "replaced" by a look-alike. He called the police and asked for their help to solve the "kidnapping." His academic performance in school declined dramatically, and he was asked to leave and seek psychiatric care.

Mr. Simpson got a job as an investment counselor at a bank, which he held for 7 months. However, he was getting an increasing number of distracting "signals" from coworkers, and he became more and more suspicious and withdrawn. It was at this time that he first reported hearing voices. He was eventually fired, and soon thereafter was hospitalized for the first time, at age 24. He has not worked since.

Mr. Simpson has been hospitalized 12 times, the longest stay being 8 months. However, in the last 5 years he has been hospitalized only once, for 3 weeks. During the hospitalizations he has received various antipsychotic drugs. Although outpatient medication has been prescribed, he usually stops taking it shortly after leaving the hospital. Aside from twice-yearly lunch meetings with his uncle and his contacts with mental health workers, he is totally isolated socially. He lives on his own and manages his own financial affairs, including a modest inheritance. He reads the *Wall Street Journal* daily. He cooks and cleans for himself.

Mr. Simpson maintains that his apartment is the center of a large communication system that involves all the major television networks, his neighbors, and apparently hundreds of "actors" in his neighborhood. There are secret cameras in his apartment that carefully monitor all his activities. When he is watching TV, many of his minor actions (e.g., going to the bathroom) are soon directly commented on by the announcer. Whenever he goes outside, the "actors" have all been warned to keep him under surveillance. Mr. Simpson states that everyone on the street watches him. He says that his neighbors operate two different "machines." One machine generates all of his voices (except the voice of the "joker"; he is uncertain who controls this voice, which "visits" him only occasionally and is very funny). He hears the voices from the machine many times each day, and he sometimes thinks the machine is directly run by the elderly neighbor whom he attacked. When he is going over his investments, the "harassing" voices from this machine constantly tell him which stocks to buy. The other machine he calls "the dream machine." This machine puts erotic dreams into his head, usually of "black women."

Mr. Simpson describes other unusual experiences. For example, he recently went to a shoe store 30 miles from his house in the hope of getting some shoes that wouldn't be "altered." However, he soon found out that, like the rest of the shoes he buys, special nails had been put into the bottom of the shoes to annoy him. He was amazed that his decision concerning which shoe store to go to must have been known to his "harassers" before he himself knew it, so that they had time to get the altered shoes made up especially for him. He realizes that great effort and "millions of dollars" are involved in keeping him under surveillance. He sometimes thinks this is all part of a large experiment to discover the secret of his "superior intelligence."

At the interview, Mr. Simpson is well-groomed, and his speech is coherent and goal-directed. His affect is, at most, only mildly blunted. He was initially very angry at being brought in by the police. After several weeks of treatment with an antipsychotic drug failed to control his psychotic symptoms, he was transferred to a long-stay facility with the plan to arrange a structured living situation for him.

SCID-5-CV Rating for "Under Surveillance"

Module A	Item Label, Rating, and Notes
Page 10:	A1 = "—"; A2 = "—"
Page 13:	A15 = "—"; A16 = "—"
Page 17:	A29 = "—"
Page 22:	A54 = "—"
Page 29:	A78 = "—"

Module B — Item Label, Rating, and Notes

Page 31: B1 = "+" (TV comments on his behavior; everyone in the street watches him; shoes are "altered" to annoy him)

B2 = "+" (machine-generated voices harass him)

Page 32: B3 = "+" ("millions of dollars" being spent, perhaps part of a large experiment to discover the secret of his "superior intelligence")

B4–B7 = "—"

Page 33: B8 = "—"

B9 = "+" (machine puts erotic dreams of "black women" in his head)

B10–B13 = "—"

B14 = "+" (machine-generated harassing voices every day)

Page 34: B15–B20 = "—"

Page 35: B21–B22 = "—"

Page 36: B23–B24 = "—"

Module C — Item Label, Rating, and Notes

Page 37: C1 = "YES" (psychotic symptoms outside of mood episodes)

C2 = "YES" (delusions and hallucinations occurring together for at least 1 month)

C3 = "YES" (no mood episode ever)

Page 38: C4 = "YES" (continuous signs of illness for years)

C5 = "YES" (marked functional impairment)

C6 = "YES" (not due to a GMC or substance/medication)

Page 44: C25 = "+" (symptoms present at some point during past month)

On the Diagnostic Summary Score Sheet, the "Current" box preceding F20.9 Schizophrenia should be checked.

SCID-5-CV diagnosis: Schizophrenia

Homework Case 6: "Agitated Businessman"

Mr. Murray, an agitated 42-year-old married white businessman, was admitted to the psychiatric service after a 2½-month period in which he found himself becoming increasingly distrustful of others and suspicious of his business associates. He was taking their statements out of context, "twisting" their words, and making inappropriately hostile and accusatory comments. He had, in fact, lost several business deals that had been "virtually sealed." Finally, the patient fired a shotgun into his backyard late one night when he heard noises that convinced him that intruders were about to break into his house and kill him.

One and one-half years previously, Mr. Murray had been diagnosed with Narcolepsy because of daily irresistible sleep attacks and episodes of sudden loss of muscle tone when he got emotionally excited. He had been placed on an amphetamine-like stimulant, methylphenidate. He became asymptomatic and was able to work quite effectively as the sales manager of a small office-machine company and to participate in an active social life with his family and a small circle of friends.

In the 4 months before admission, he had been using increasingly large doses of methylphenidate to maintain alertness late at night because of an increasing amount of work that could not be handled during the day. He reported that during this time he often could feel his heart race and had trouble sitting still.

SCID-5-CV Rating for "Agitated Businessman"

Module A	Item Label, Rating, and Notes
Page 10:	A1 = "—"; A2 = "—"
Page 13:	A15 = "—"; A16 = "—"
Page 17:	A29 = "—"
Page 22:	A54 = "—"
Page 29:	A78 = "—"

Module B	Item Label, Rating, and Notes
Page 31:	B1 = "+" (he heard noises that convinced him that intruders were about to break into his house and kill him)
	B2 = "+" (suspicious of business associates, but not clear that he has a delusional conviction about any particular issue; remember to give the patient the benefit of the doubt when a psychotic symptom is not clearly present)
Page 32:	B3–B7 = "—"
Page 33:	B8–B13 = "—"
	B14 = "—" (noises he heard outside are more likely to have been misinterpreted than to be true hallucinations)
Page 34:	B15–B20 = "—"
Page 35:	B21–B22 = "—"
Page 36:	B23–B24 = "—"

Module C	Item Label, Rating, and Notes
Page 37:	C1 = "YES" (psychotic symptoms outside of mood episodes)
	C2 = "NO" (only delusion of reference)
Page 40:	C13 = "YES" (delusions for 2 months)
	C14 = "YES" (has not met Criterion A for Schizophrenia)
	C15 = "YES" (behavior not markedly impaired or bizarre)
Page 41:	C16 = "YES" (no Manic or Major Depressive Episodes)
	C17 = "NO" (due to a substance/medication)
	On the Diagnostic Summary Score Sheet, the "Lifetime" box for Substance/Medication-Induced Psychotic Disorder should be checked. The specific substance (Adderall) and the ICD-10-CM diagnostic code, F15.959, should also be recorded.

SCID-5-CV diagnosis: Substance/Medication-Induced Psychotic Disorder

Homework Case 7: "Bad Voices"

Ms. Galvez is an attractive, 25-year-old divorced Dominican mother of two children. A redhead with a pouty and seductive demeanor, Ms. Galvez was referred to the psychiatric emergency room by a psychiatrist who was treating her in an anxiety disorders clinic. After telling her doctor that she heard voices telling her to kill herself, and then assuring him that she would not act on the voices, Ms. Galvez skipped her next appointment. Her doctor called her to say that if she did not voluntarily come to the emergency room for an evaluation, he would send the police for her.

Interviewed in the emergency room by a senior psychiatrist with a group of emergency room psychiatric residents, Ms. Galvez was at times angry and insistent that she did not like to talk about her problems, and that the psychiatrists would not believe her or help her anyway. This attitude alternated with flirtatious and seductive behavior.

Ms. Galvez first saw a psychiatrist 7 years previously, after the birth of her first child. At that time, she began to hear a voice telling her that she was a bad person and that she should kill herself. She would not say exactly what it told her to do, but she reportedly drank nail polish remover in a suicide attempt. At that time, she remained in the emergency room for 2 days and received an unknown medication that reportedly helped quiet the voices. She did not return for an outpatient appointment after discharge, and continued having intermittent periods of auditory hallucinations at various points over the next 7 years, with some periods lasting for months at a time. For example, often when she was near a window, a voice would tell her to jump out; and when she walked near traffic, it would tell her to walk in front of a car.

She reports that she continued to function well after that first episode, finishing high school and raising her children. She was divorced a year ago, but she refused to discuss her marital problems. About 2 months ago, she began to have trouble sleeping and felt "nervous." It was at this time that she responded to an ad for the anxiety disorders clinic. She was evaluated and given risperidone, an antipsychotic. She claims that there was no change in the voices at that time, and only the insomnia and anxiety were new. She specifically denied depressed mood or anhedonia, or any change in her appetite, but did report that she was more tearful and lonely, and sometimes ruminated about "bad things," such as her father's attempted rape of her at age 14. Despite these symptoms, she continued working more than full-time as a salesperson in a department store.

Ms. Galvez says she did not keep her follow-up appointment at the anxiety disorders clinic because the risperidone was making her stiff and nauseated and was not helping her symptoms. She denies wanting to kill herself, and cites how hard she is working to raise her children as evidence that she would not "leave them that way." She did not understand why her behavior had alarmed her psychiatrist.

Ms. Galvez denied alcohol or drug use, and a toxicology screen for various drugs was negative. Physical examination and routine laboratory tests were also normal. She had stopped the risperidone on her own 2 days before the interview.

Following the interview, there was disagreement among the staff about whether to let the patient leave. It was finally decided to keep her overnight, until her mother could be interviewed the next day. When told she was to stay in the emergency room, she replied angrily, yet somewhat coyly: "Go ahead. You'll have to let me out sooner or later, but I don't have to talk to you if I don't want to." During the night, nursing staff noticed that she was tearful, but she said she didn't know why she was crying.

When her mother was interviewed the following morning, she said she did not see a recent change in her daughter. She did not feel that her daughter would hurt herself, but agreed to stay with her for a few days and make sure she went for follow-up appointments. In the family meeting, Ms. Galvez complained that her mother was unresponsive and did not help her enough. However, she again denied depression and said she enjoyed her job and her children. About the voices, she said that over time she had learned how to ignore them, and that they did not bother her as much as they had at first. She agreed to outpatient treatment provided the therapist was a female.

SCID-5-CV Rating for "Bad Voices"

Module A	Item Label, Rating, and Notes
Page 10:	A1 = "—"; A2 = "—"
Page 13:	A15 = "—"; A16 = "—"
Page 17:	A29 = "—"
Page 22:	A54 = "—"
Page 29:	A78 = "—"

Module B	Item Label, Rating, and Notes
Page 31:	B1–B2 = "—"
Page 32:	B3–B7 = "—"
Page 33:	B8–B13 = "—"
	B14 = "+" (voices telling her she's a bad person and to kill herself)
Page 34:	B15–B20 = "—"
Page 35:	B21–B22 = "—"
Page 36:	B23–B24 = "—"

Module C	Item Label, Rating, and Notes
Page 37:	C1 = "YES" (no documentation of mood episodes)
	C2 = "NO" (hallucinations only)
Page 40:	C13 = "NO" (never any delusions)
Page 41:	C19 = "YES" (hallucinations)
Page 42:	C20 = "NO" (hallucinations lasted more than 1 month)
	C22 = "YES" (does not meet full criteria for other psychotic disorders)
	C23 = "YES" (causes impairment)
Page 43:	C24 = "YES" (not due to a GMC or substance/medication)
Page 44:	C30 = "+" (symptoms present at some point during past month)

On the Diagnostic Summary Score Sheet, the "Current" box preceding F28 Other Specified Schizophrenia Spectrum and Other Psychotic Disorder should be checked and the description of the presentation ("persistent auditory hallucinations") should be recorded.

SCID-5-CV diagnosis: Other Specified Psychotic Disorder

Homework Case 8: "Late Bloomer"

Ms. Fielding is a 35-year-old single, unemployed, college-educated African American woman who was escorted to the emergency room by the mobile crisis team. The team had been contacted by Ms. Fielding's sister after she had failed to persuade Ms. Fielding to visit an outpatient psychiatrist. The sister was concerned about Ms. Fielding's increasingly erratic work pattern and, more recently, bizarre behavior since the death of their father 2 years ago. Ms. Fielding's only prior psychiatric contact had been brief psychotherapy in college.

Ms. Fielding has not worked since being laid off from her job 3 months ago. According to her boyfriend and roommate (both of whom live with her), she became intensely preoccupied with the upstairs neighbors. A few days ago, she banged on their front door with an iron for no apparent reason. She told the mobile crisis team that the family upstairs was harassing her by "accessing" her thoughts and then repeating them to her. The crisis team brought her to the emergency room for evaluation of "thought broadcasting." Though she denied having any trouble with her thinking, she conceded that she was feeling "stressed" since losing her job and might benefit from more psychotherapy.

After reading the admission note that described such bizarre symptoms, the emergency room psychiatrists were surprised to encounter a poised, relaxed, and attractive young woman, stylishly dressed and appearing perfectly normal. She greeted them with a courteous, if somewhat superficial, smile. She related to the doctors with nonchalant respectfulness. When asked why she was there, she ventured a timid shrug, and replied, "I was hoping to find out from you!"

Ms. Fielding had been working as a secretary and attributed her job loss to the sluggish economy. She said she was "stressed out" by her unemployment. She denied having any recent mood disturbance, and answered "NO" to questions about psychotic symptoms, punctuating each query with a polite but incredulous laugh. Wondering if perhaps the crisis team's assessment was of a different patient, the interviewer asked, somewhat apologetically, if Ms. Fielding ever wondered whether people could read her mind. She replied, "Oh yes, it happens all the time," and described how, on one occasion, she was standing in her kitchen planning dinner in silence only to hear, moments later, voices of people on the street below reciting the entire menu. She was convinced of the reality of the experience, having verified it by looking out the window and observing them speaking her thoughts aloud.

Ms. Fielding was distressed not so much by people "accessing" her thoughts as by her inability to exercise control over the process. She believed that most people developed telepathic powers in childhood, while she was a "late bloomer" who had just become aware of her abilities, and was currently overwhelmed by them. She was troubled mostly by her upstairs neighbors, who would not only repeat her thoughts but also bombard her with their own devaluing and critical comments, such as "You're no good" and "You have to leave." They had begun to intrude upon her mercilessly, at all hours of the night and day.

She was convinced that the only solution was for the family to move away. When asked if she had contemplated other possibilities, she reluctantly admitted that she had spoken to her boyfriend about hiring a hit man to "threaten" or, if need be, "eliminate" the couple. She hoped she would be able to spare their two children, whom she felt were not involved in this invasion of her "mental boundaries." This concern for the children was the only insight she demonstrated into the gravity of her symptoms. She did agree, however, to admit herself voluntarily to the hospital.

SCID-5-CV Rating for "Late Bloomer"

Module A	Item Label, Rating, and Notes
Page 10:	A1 = "—"; A2 = "—"
Page 13:	A15 = "—"; A16 = "—"
Page 17:	A29 = "—"
Page 22:	A54 = "—"
Page 29:	A78 = "—"

Module B	Item Label, Rating, and Notes
Page 31:	B1 = "+" (observed people on the street speaking her thoughts aloud)
	B2 = "+" (neighbors are "harassing" her)
Page 32:	B3 = "—" (her "telepathic powers" are not grandiose in content)
	B4–B7 = "—"
Page 33:	B8–B12 = "—"
	B13 = "+" (people can read her mind)
	B14 = "+" (heard voices of people on the street below reciting entire menu; voices of upstairs neighbors bombarding her with their own devaluing and critical comments, such as "You're no good" and "You have to leave")
Page 34:	B15–B20 = "—"
Page 35:	B21–B22 = "—"
Page 36:	B23–B24 = "—"

Module C	Item Label, Rating, and Notes
Page 37:	C1 = "YES" (no mood episodes)
	C2 = "YES" (delusions and hallucinations occurring together for at least 1 month)
	C3 = "YES" (no mood episode ever)
Page 38:	C4 = "NO" (psychotic symptoms for only 3 months)
Page 39:	C7 = "YES" (symptoms last at least 1 month but less than 6 months)
	C8 = "YES" (not due to a GMC or substance/medication)
Page 44:	C26 = "+" (symptoms present at some point during past month)
	On the Diagnostic Summary Score Sheet, the "Current" box preceding F20.81 Schizophreniform Disorder should be checked.

SCID-5-CV diagnosis: Schizophreniform Disorder

Homework Case 9: "Radar Messages"

Ms. Davis, a 24-year-old, single, white copyeditor who has recently moved from Colorado to New York, comes to a psychiatrist for help in continuing her treatment with a mood stabilizer, lithium. She describes how, 3 years previously, she was a successful college student in her senior year, doing well academically and enjoying a large circle of friends of both sexes. In the midst of an uneventful period in the first semester (October 2011), she began to feel depressed; experienced loss of appetite, with a weight loss of about 10 pounds; had trouble falling asleep and waking up too early; had severe fatigue, felt worthless, and had great difficulty concentrating on her schoolwork.

After about 2 months of these problems, they seemed to go away, but she then began to feel increasingly energetic, requiring only 2–3 hours of sleep at night, and to experience her thoughts as "racing." She started to see symbolic meanings in things, especially sexual meanings, and began to suspect that innocent comments on television shows were referring to her. Over the next month, she became increasingly euphoric, irritable, and overtalkative. She started to believe that there was a hole in her head through which radar messages were being sent to her. These messages could control her thoughts or produce emotions of anger, sadness, or the like, which were beyond her control. She also believed that her thoughts could be read by people around her and that alien thoughts from other people were intruding themselves via the radar into her own head. She described hearing voices, which sometimes spoke about her in the third person and at other times ordered her to perform various acts, particularly sexual ones.

Her friends, concerned about Ms. Davis's unusual behavior, took her to an emergency room, where she was evaluated and admitted to a psychiatric unit. After a day of observation, Ms. Davis was started on an antipsychotic, olanzapine, and lithium carbonate. Over the course of about 3 weeks, she experienced a fairly rapid reduction in all of the symptoms that had brought her to the hospital. The olanzapine was gradually reduced, and then discontinued. She was maintained thereafter on lithium carbonate alone. At the time of her discharge, after 6 weeks of hospitalization, she was exhibiting none of the symptoms reported on admission. However, she was noted to be experiencing some mild hypersomnia, sleeping about 10 hours a night; loss of appetite; and some feeling of being "slowed down," which was worse in the mornings. She was discharged to live with some friends.

Approximately 8 months after her discharge, Ms. Davis was taken off lithium carbonate by the psychiatrist in the college mental health clinic. She continued to do fairly well for the next few months, but then began to experience a gradual reappearance of symptoms similar to those that had necessitated her hospitalization. The symptoms worsened, and after 2 weeks she was readmitted to the hospital with almost the identical symptoms that she had when first admitted.

Ms. Davis responded in days to olanzapine and lithium; and once again, the olanzapine was gradually discontinued, leaving her on lithium alone. As with the first hospitalization, at the time of her discharge, a little more than 1 year ago, she again displayed some hypersomnia, loss of appetite, and the feeling of being "slowed down." For the past year, while continuing to take lithium, she has been symptom free and functioning fairly well, getting a job in publishing and recently moving to New York to advance her career.

Ms. Davis's father, when in his 40s, had had a severe episode of depression, characterized by hypersomnia, anorexia, profound psychomotor retardation, and suicidal ideation. Her paternal grandmother had committed suicide during what also appeared to be a depressive episode.

SCID-5-CV Rating for "Radar Messages"

Module A	Item Label, Rating, and Notes
Page 10:	A1 = "—"; A2 = "—"
Page 13:	A15 = "+" (3 years ago, began to feel depressed)
	A16 = "—"
Page 14:	A17 = "+" (loss of appetite; 10-pound weight loss)
	A18 = "+" (trouble falling asleep; waking up too early)
	A19 = "—"
	A20 = "+" (severe fatigue)
	A21 = "+" (feelings of worthlessness)
	A22 = "+" (difficulty concentrating)
Page 15:	A23 = "+" (suicidal ideation)
	A24 = "YES" (Criterion A met for past Major Depressive Episode)
	A25 = "+" (clinically significant)
Page 16:	A26 = "YES" (not due to a GMC or substance/medication)
	A27 = "10/2011" (date of onset)
	A28 = "01" (number of episodes)
Page 17:	A29 = "—" (no current euphoric or irritable mood)
Page 22:	A54 = "+" (3 years ago, became increasingly euphoric and irritable)
Page 23:	A55 = "+" (hospitalized)
	A56 = "—"
	A57 = "+" (required only 2–3 hours of sleep a night)
	A58 = "+" (overtalkative)
	A59 = "+" (began to experience her thoughts as "racing")
	A60 = "—"
Page 24:	A61 = "—"
	A62 = "—"
	A63 = "YES" (three symptoms coded "+")
Page 25:	A64 = "+" (hospitalized)
	A65 = "+" (not due to a GMC or substance/medication)

Module B	Item Label, Rating, and Notes
Page 31:	B1 = "+" (innocent comments on television shows were referring to her)
	B2 = "—" (no clear malevolent intent of radar messages)
Page 32:	B3 = "—"
	B4 = "+" ("hole in her head")
	B5–B7 = "—"
Page 33:	B8 = "—"
	B9 = "+" (radar messages could control her thoughts)
	B10 = "+"(alien thoughts from other people were intruding themselves)
	B11–B12 = "—"
	B13 = "+" (believed her thoughts could be read by other people around her)
	B14 = "+" (heard voices)
Page 34:	B15–B20 = "—"
Page 35:	B21–B22 = "—"
Page 36:	B23–B24 = "—"

Module C	Item Label, Rating, and Notes
Page 37:	C1 = "NO" (psychotic symptoms only during Manic Episodes)

Module D	Item Label, Rating, and Notes
Page 45:	D2 = "YES" (Manic Episodes)
	D3 = "YES" (not explained by Psychotic Disorder), "1" (Most Recent Episode Manic)
Page 49:	D17 = "—" (no symptoms in past 2 months)
	On the Diagnostic Summary Score Sheet, the "Past History" box preceding F31.74 Bipolar I Disorder, Most Recent Episode Manic, In Full Remission, should be checked.

**SCID-5-CV diagnosis: Bipolar I Disorder, Most Recent Episode Manic,
                          In Full Remission**